Needs and Capacity Assessment Strategies for Health Education and Health Promotion

THIRD EDITION

Gary D. Gilmore, MPH, PhD, CHES

Professor and Director
Community Health Programs
University of Wisconsin–La Crosse and
University of Wisconsin–Extension

M. Donald Campbell, PhD

Director
Continuing Education and Extension
University of Wisconsin–La Crosse

JONES AND BARTLETT PUBLISHERS
Sudbury, Massachusetts
BOSTON   TORONTO   LONDON   SINGAPORE

World Headquarters
Jones and Bartlett Publishers
40 Tall Pine Drive
Sudbury, MA 01776
978-443-5000
info@jbpub.com
www.jbpub.com

Jones and Bartlett
  Publishers Canada
6339 Ormindale Way
Mississauga,
  ON L5V 1J2
CANADA

Jones and Bartlett
  Publishers
  International
Barb House, Barb Mews
London W6 7PA
UK

ISBN-13: 978-0-7637-2599-0
ISBN-10: 0-7637-2599-4

Production Credits
Acquisitions Editor: Jacqueline Ann Mark
Production Editor: Julie Champagne Bolduc
Associate Editor: Nicole Quinn
Marketing Manager: Ed McKenna
Director of Interactive Technology: Adam Alboyadjian
Manufacturing Buyer: Therese Connell
Photo Researcher: Kimberly Potvin
Composition: Interactive Composition Corporation
Cover Design: Anne Spencer
Cover Images: (background) © AbleStock; (left to right) © John A. Rizzo/ Photodisc/Getty
    Images, © Adrian Arbib/Alamy Images, © Veer, © Robert Harding World Imagery/Alamy
    Images
Printing and Binding: Malloy, Inc.
Cover Printing: Malloy, Inc.

Library of Congress Cataloging-in-Publication Data
Gilmore, Gary D., 1943-
  Needs and capacity assessment strategies for health education and health
    promotion / Gary D. Gilmore, M. Donald Campbell.— 3rd ed.
      p. ; cm.
  Rev. ed. of: Needs assessment strategies for health education and health
    promotion. 1996.
  Includes bibliographical references and index.
  ISBN 0-7637-2599-4
1. Medical personnel—Supply and demand. 2. Public health personnel—Supply and demand.
3. Health promotion—Evaluation.
  [DNLM: 1. Health Services Research—methods. 2. Health Education—organization &
administration. 3. Health Promotion—organization & administration. 4. Health Services
Needs and Demand. W 84.3 G486n 2005] I. Campbell, M. Donald. II. Gilmore, Gary D.,
1943- Needs assessment strategies for health education and health promotion. III. Title.
  RA440.4.G55 2005
    362.1'0723—dc22
6048   2004003773

Printed in the United States of America
10 09 08 07 06 10 9 8 7 6 5 4 3 2

*For John and Ruth; Elizabeth, Scott, Todd, and Merrily,
for always being there.*

For Louise, David, and Andrew.

Contents

Part V Case Studies and a Needs Assessment Simulation   165

Case Study Descriptions

Appendices

Foreword

As in their previous editions, Gilmore and Campbell have captured the essence of the demand of practitioners for practical tools and the growing literature on methods and measures for assessment of needs. They have added in this edition a complementary set of tools and methods for assessment of capacity. Their combination of needs assessment and capacity assessment strategies provides practitioners with the right balance for formative evaluation and planning with community leaders who are cynical about another round of needs assessment that fails to acknowledge the strengths and assets of the community. Capacity assessment offers an antidote to the despair that comes with identifying one's community problems. All too often, such needs assessments go to the academic press or, even worse, to the popular press, to the chagrin and embarrassment of the community. All too often, those who publish findings about community needs fail to offer help—let alone solutions—to address the needs identified. Leaving the community with at least an inventory of its assets and capacity gives its leaders a foundation of pride and resources for tackling their problems.

In Chapter 1, the authors cast their methods in the broader context of skills required for professional performance. In Chapter 2, they cast needs and capacity development in the broader context of program planning. As authors of a book on program planning, my co-author Marshall Kreuter and I are indebted to Gilmore and Campbell for the pressure their book takes off of us to provide much of the detailed description and procedures of some of the needs and capacity assessment steps in planning that this book provides. Even if we thought we could do it as well, we would be ill advised to repeat much of what is now so well presented and documented in this book.

In Chapters 3 through 9, Gilmore and Campbell give the detailed description and procedures for applying each of the major methods of data collection for needs and capacity assessment. In Chapter 10, they outline the large-scale assessment strategies, including emerging community-based assessment procedures such as APEX-PH, COMPASS, MAPP, and PATCH. Finally, they offer self-assessment inventories and appraisals, and early detection procedures.

These variations on the methods of needs and capacity assessment should give the busy practitioner the menu of options to find the right fit for his or her own community assessment and planning circumstances.

Lawrence W. Green, DrPH
Director, Office of Science and Extramural Research
Public Health Practice Program Office
Centers for Disease Control and Prevention
U.S. Department of Health and Human Services
Atlanta, Georgia

Preface

More health professionals are involved in needs and capacity assessment strategies today than ever before. A variety of reasons explain this trend: an increased desire to be as cost-effective as possible; an increased emphasis on the use of marketing strategies with identified target groups; a focus on accountability for the time and financial commitments made by health professionals; rising consumer demand for health services that truly meet consumer needs, rather than taking a "one size fits all" approach; and an emerging emphasis on participating with community members in the development and implementation of health education and health promotional research and intervention activities.

Our purpose for writing this third edition was to update all of the strategies included in the first two editions, address emerging issues in capacity-focused assessments and community empowerment issues, and add to the chapter examples, case studies, and appendices. In the process, we continued to address the alignment of the needs and capacity strategies with already-established planning frameworks, particularly the PRECEDE-PROCEED approach.

In this edition, we retain our focus on reviewing realistic needs and capacity assessment strategies with considerations for preparation, implementation, and incorporation of the findings into the planning process. As in the first two editions, examples are provided at the end of each chapter based on our experiences and those of others. Additionally, we continue to offer expanded examples of various combinations of strategies used in a variety of settings through the discussions in the case studies. These provide an overview of the settings, specific target audiences, approaches to assessing needs, and handling of any problems encountered along the way. Actual assessment inventory examples have been updated and included in the case studies and appendices.

We continue with our efforts to have this text be a reader-friendly sourcebook of ideas and practical strategies. For this reason, you will note our attempts to include needs and capacity assessment strategies that can be infused into one's current professional responsibilities rather easily.

With a project of this magnitude, many individuals inevitably take part. We fully appreciate the thoughtful insights shared by Dr. Lawrence Green in his Foreword to this book, as he draws from his decades of experience in health education and health promotion research and practice. Others who have made important contributions to this third edition are Cynthia Currence, Harmon Eyre, Robert Gorsky, Jill Hubbard, Elaine Jones, Donell Kerns, Douglas Mormann, Larry Olsen, Kathy Olson, Kay Robinson, Megan Sheffer, Larry Sleznikow, Robert Smith, and Terry Wirkus. We wish to acknowledge those on the Editorial and Health Development Team at Jones and Bartlett with whom we have communicated during the development of this project: Kris Ellis, former Health Acquisitions Editor; Jacqueline Mark, Acquisitions Editor for Health and Nutrition Titles; Julie Bolduc, Production Editor; Nicole Quinn, Associate Editor; and Ed McKenna, Marketing Manager.

Gary D. Gilmore
M. Donald Campbell

About the Authors

Gary D. Gilmore, MPH, PhD, CHES

Since 1974, Dr. Gilmore has held a joint appointment with the University of Wisconsin–La Crosse and the University of Wisconsin–Extension. He is Professor and Director of Community Health Programs. His prior experiences have been in public health and preventive medicine at the Bergen County Department (New Jersey), and at the Preventive Medicine Unit, General Leonard Wood Hospital, U.S. Army (where he was the recipient of the Army Commendation Medal in Preventive Medicine). Dr. Gilmore received his training in epidemiology and public health education at the School of Public Health at the University of Minnesota, with additional training in epidemiology at the New England Epidemiology Institute, Tufts University.

Dr. Gilmore is the founding and continuing Director of the first Master of Public Health Program (CEPH accredited) offered in the University of Wisconsin System. As an inherent part of his appointment, he directs the Community Health Programming Unit in Continuing Education and Extension (University of Wisconsin–Extension). He served on the American Cancer Society National Board of Directors during the 1986–1996 and 1999–2002 periods, and is the recipient of that organization's St. George Medal for "outstanding contributions to the control of cancer." Dr. Gilmore received the 2001 Regents Teaching Excellence Award bestowed by the Board of Regents, University of Wisconsin System. He also received the 1998 Award for Excellence from the University of Wisconsin–Extension.

During 1999–2000, Dr. Gilmore served as the first Fulbright Senior Scholar at the All India Institute of Hygiene and Public Health in Calcutta, India. In that capacity, he taught graduate students and medical students in public health, and conducted population-based research in West Bengal.

Dr. Gilmore's publications span more than three decades of professional activity and include peer-reviewed journal articles, books, and technical reports. He currently chairs the six-year National Health Educator Competencies Update Project, which seeks to validate the entry- and advanced-level competencies for health education specialists. The results of this national research will affect advancements in professional preparation, credentialing, and professional development.

M. Donald Campbell, PhD
Dr. Campbell is Director of the Office of Continuing Education and Extension, University of Wisconsin–La Crosse. He oversees the delivery of off-campus credit programs, as well as conferences, workshops, and other noncredit programs for health and human service professionals, other professional audiences, and community groups. Previously, he was Director, Continuing Medical Education for the University of Illinois College of Medicine at Urbana-Champaign.

Dr. Campbell has taught graduate courses in continuing education and program development, and served as book review editor for *Continuing Higher Education Review*. He has conducted needs assessments and program evaluations for a variety of professional audiences. His research focuses on the impact of continuing education on professional practice.

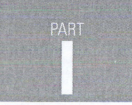

Introduction and Overview

In Chapters 1 and 2 we present emerging and established key issues related to needs, resources, and needs and capacity assessments, and we consider how they fit into the larger framework of planning for health education and health promotion. In addition, we address a variety of preliminary considerations for health and human service professionals, including a review of capacity-focused assessments, advisory and planning committees, community coalitions, selected data collection considerations, and prioritization processes. All of these elements, including a statement of our basic premises, form a context within which the selected needs and capacity assessment strategies are employed.

Gaining a Needs and Capacity Assessment Perspective

Introduction

Trends

On September 11, 2001, terrorists attacked and destroyed the World Trade Center in New York City, killing an estimated 2,819 persons (CDC, 2002). In the wake of this disaster, surveys were developed to gather information regarding physical and psychological impacts so as to establish priorities and direct public health intervention strategies. Door-to-door interviews (CDC, 2002) and telephone interviews (Galea, Ahern, and Resnick, 2002) were used to make the assessments regarding incidence of post-traumatic stress disorder (PTSD), incidence of physical ailments, availability of household utility services, need for information about hazards related to dust and debris exposure, proper cleaning procedures, and availability of mental health and relief services. Of particular note, it was projected that about 87,000 people in Manhattan needed mental health services, and about 67,000 needed services for PTSD. In addition to the obvious galvanizing effect this incident had on the nation as a whole, needs and capacity assessments were important components in the disaster response.

During instances of almost any magnitude of impact, having health-related assessments in place promotes the systematic and timely review of requisite resources. Toward the end of the last century, and continuing into the twenty-first century, needs and capacity assessments have become more prominent procedures within health education and health promotion planning, and other planning endeavors as well. This amplification is happening with good reason. Insights into health-related impacts on a society are ever expanding in terms of their *nature* (e.g., the interactivity of physical, psychological, and behavioral factors related to disease risk), *degree* (e.g., poverty's impact on health outcomes), and *setting* (e.g., the global impacts of violent behavior), thus necessitating consistent, systematic assessment principles and practices. Additionally, accountability issues increase as resources become scarcer, leading to calls for more evidence-based endeavors. Furthermore, within the rubric of "workforce development," professional competencies need to be ascertained and periodically validated in health education, health promotion, and even the broader context of public health, requiring greater specificity of professional skill sets.

Specifically for health education, one of the key areas of responsibility for entry-level and advanced-level health educators is the assessment of individual and community needs for health education (NCHEC, 1996; AAHE, NCHEC, and SOPHE, 1999). Included in this responsibility area are the aspects of obtaining health-related data, distinguishing between behaviors that enhance well-being and behaviors that impede well-being, and inferring needs for health education. More recent national competency validation research (Gilmore, Olsen, and Taub, 2001) demonstrates the importance of revalidating established competencies, and verifying the existence of additional competencies that have emerged in the profession.

In similar fashion, practitioners in other disciplines are recognizing the value of needs and capacity assessments as integral parts of the planning process. As one example, some business professionals involved in worksite health promotion are recommending frameworks that incorporate clearly identified needs and capacity assessments so that objective information can be collected to guide the next steps in the planning process. Bensky and Hietbrink (1994) have described a health promotion planning framework for business settings (to be discussed in greater detail in Chapter 2) in which they state that "most health promotion programs that fail to reach their goals are built upon invalid assumptions about what people need, want and will do about it" (p. 26). They then detail the first step in their planning framework, which is assessing the situation. Assessments at the worksite setting can also be quite comprehensive, as described by Oldenburg and colleagues (2002) through their 112-item checklist of workplace environmental factors that affect health enhancement both negatively and positively. Their assessment categories include a building assessment, the information environment (e.g., signs and bulletin boards), fitness facilities, grounds and neighborhood assessments, and assessments of various individual-choice practices related to nutrition, smoking, and alcohol activities at the worksite.

To track some of the patterns regarding needs and capacity assessments that have emerged during the last decade, we must recognize the changes noted below.

First, needs and capacity assessments are being incorporated into various professional responsibilities to a greater extent. More professionals are using these assessments as inherent parts of their work in public health departments, hospitals, clinics, schools, voluntary and other private agencies, and business sites. This shift appears to be due to a greater emphasis on documentation to justify programs and initiatives and their costs, as well as the increased use of marketing strategies to address target population needs and resources in school, community, and business settings. Also, cost-conscious consumers are becoming more selective in their health-related choices, based to a large extent on a desire to have specific needs met at a reasonable cost. From a capacity perspective, community-based groups appreciate being recognized as resources that can be drawn upon during the planning, implementation, and evaluation of health education and health promotional activities. In response, health program and service providers have shown a renewed interest in ascertaining the needs and capacities, as revealed by the consumers. All of these aspects— documentation, marketing strategies, and program and service offerings— typically drive the use of needs assessments as a starting point for determining specific population needs. The results can guide more effective planning and implementation strategies. Additionally, capacity assessment procedures have been expanded in the planning process to explore existing and needed resources in school, community, and business settings.

A second change has to do with the broader context of the "needs" being assessed. Here we refer to factors that influence health status, to include risk factors, protective factors (sometimes referred to as assets), and a wide range of determinants that constitute a context of influence on the health status of individuals and communities. These determinants include biological, behavioral, and social influences, as defined and delineated in a 2001 report by the Institute of Medicine (IOM), and as incorporated into *Healthy People 2010* (USDHHS, 2000). Throughout this text, while specific examples of needs will be provided, it is most important for health and human service professionals to keep this more comprehensive perspective in mind.

Third, we have noted an emergence of individualized assessment strategies. These personal approaches can be quite valuable in health maintenance and health promotional efforts (see Chapters 11 and 12). They can enable a person to detect specific risk factors that may negatively affect his or her own health. Individualized capacity assessment strategies also can help a person identify other factors and resources that are quite positive and enhance good health in the individual's life.

A fourth change is the wide variance in what is meant by "needs assessment" and "capacity assessment," and how these terms are used. Regarding needs assessments, there is much discussion as to what a "need" is, and whether we assess actual or perceived needs. Health and human service professionals have different reasons for using this process. Some professionals use needs assessments as starting points for program planning. Others use them on a continuing basis with the same populations to detect changing needs over a certain period of time, and to adjust the services based on those needs. Similarly, in addressing "capacity assessment," ascertaining actual and potential resources can contribute to more efficient planning, in preparing to use available and emerging population-based resources to complement external wherewithal.

This approach also can result in meta-benefits, such as the involved individu. having a greater sense of feeling valued as contributors, thereby resulting i increased commitment to a project or initiative.

Fifth, community-based participatory approaches to research and practice have emerged to address the social determinants of health in particular (Schulz, Krieger, and Galea, 2002). As Schulz et al. (2002) point out, risk factors explain only a portion of outcomes such as coronary heart disease, because the risks themselves can be affected by more contextual factors such as poverty, discrimination, education, and housing policies. To address these complexities, collaborative and innovative research and intervention strategies are required, necessitating the awareness and involvement of community members in organized research and intervention strategies. This awareness by health and human service professionals and community members has led to the emergence of community-based participatory approaches in which community members become involved in the essential phases of project planning, implementation, and evaluation.

Sixth, as an inherent part of community-based assessment activity, it is increasingly important to work in partnership with the community, rather than viewing it as a setting in which professionals conduct investigations known only to them. The Office of Disease Prevention and Health Promotion, which is part of the U.S. Public Health Service (2001), has called for more of a collaborative endeavor, viewing communities as cornerstones of public health action, and offering a planning guide to be discussed in more detail in Chapter 10. Corroborating this perspective, the 2003 Institute of Medicine report, *Who Will Keep the Public Healthy?*, has addressed the value and importance of community-based research, in which key community rep-resentatives become engaged in the development and implementation of such investigations. Israel et al. (2001) have defined community-based participatory research as a "partnership approach to research that equitably involves community members, organizational representatives, and researchers in all aspects of the research process" (p. 2). Miller, Bedney, and Guenther-Grey (2003) have emphasized the degree to which collaborative efforts can facilitate community-wide change. As they point out, "collaborative work highlights the role of community systems and the interdependence among community sectors in affecting health outcomes" (p. 583). To collaborate effectively, they point to the importance of all partners sharing a clear mission and plan centered on mutual goals. The importance of community involvement is conveyed in federal requests for proposals (RFPs), such as the comprehensive *HealthierUS* approach to prevention in the United States (CDC, 2003), which calls for a formal assessment of community needs and assets, in addition to the usual project development processes of planning, delivery, and evaluation (see the Federal Register, May 9, 2003). Additional information about the *HealthierUS* effort can be found at http://www.healthierUS.gov.

continuing emphasis on capacity analysis to complement ~ process. As Kretzmann and McKnight (1993) have ~apacity-focused approach addresses the capacities, skills, and ~ a community. Through this approach, which will be covered in more ~tail in Chapter 2, the assets of a community are mapped by examining the potential contributions of individuals, organizations, associations, and institutions. In the years following the insights first provided by Kretzmann and McKnight (1993), capacity-building approaches to community health promotion have been more widely embraced and incorporated into systematic planning efforts, including school health promotion efforts (Bond, Glover, Godfrey, et al., 2001).

Eighth, large-scale community assessment formats have appeared on the scene, providing comprehensive direction to planners seeking organizational and community assessments. The Assessment Protocol for Excellence in Public Health (APEX-PH) is one such format and will be discussed in greater detail in Chapter 10 (Pratt, McDonald, Libby, et al., 1996). These frameworks use a variety of assessment approaches that draw upon previously gathered information (secondary data), while preparing to collect additional information from the target population (primary data).

Ninth, needs and capacity assessments are being incorporated into emergency circumstances where there is an urgency in assessing human needs and the capacity to assure health and well-being. The response to the World Trade Center attack described earlier is just one example. Another example is the assessment measures taken following the major earthquake that struck Turkey in 1999 (Daley, Karpati, and Sheik, 2002). Preparation for future emergency circumstances is an imperative for community planning measures regarding the roles of health care, public health, and human service professionals, along with the needed communication technology and content appropriate for both professionals and the public (Taintor, 2003).

Key Questions about Assessment

Whether one is a health or human service professional just beginning employment, or someone with considerable experience, the meaning and processes of needs and capacity assessment can appear to be quite confounding. The following questions represent those we hear most frequently. For the sake of clarification, we offer preliminary responses to them.

What is a need? A need is the difference between the present situation and a more desirable one. The present situation may have some undesirable characteristics that motivate one to consider a more desirable situation. For example, we might realize that we are overweight and "need" to identify the causes and ways to resolve the problem. But needs are not solely related to undesirable situations; a very positive situation can be further enhanced. For example, you might jog two miles every other day to keep fit, and want to increase the distance. Or, you might have learned to avoid some of the risk factors related to cancer (e.g., smoking), and now want to learn more about protective factors against cancer (e.g., adding more fiber to your diet).

What is a needs assessment? A needs assessment is a planned process that identifies the reported needs of an individual or a group. Individuals can conduct needs assessments that reveal reported areas of personal needs. A person can review these needs, consider their relative importance and practicality, and then take steps to address them. With groups, a subgroup that is representative of the larger group can work through the needs assessment process. Health professionals can use the reported needs from this representative group for planning purposes.

Are the reported needs actual or perceived? It is difficult for the health or human service professional, and even for the target audience, to know whether the needs identified by an individual or group are the actual needs (the *true* needs). These actual needs are difficult to identify and measure because they change continually. Perceived needs are those envisioned and reported by the participants in a needs assessment process (the *reported* needs). As professionals involved in a needs assessment, we rely upon people as primary sources of information. These people draw from their experiences, observations, ideas, opinions, and feelings to guide them toward conclusions about needs—perceived needs. We recognize the importance of perceived needs because they represent the experiences and perceptions of the individuals or groups involved. We believe it is inefficient to expend a great deal of energy trying to determine whether perceived needs are actual needs. Because individuals and groups are continually changing and growing, their needs are changing as well. The strategies we present do not attempt to determine true needs beyond any shadow of a doubt. Rather, our purpose is to describe workable processes that assess perceived needs of individual and group importance.

Why conduct a needs assessment? A needs assessment provides a logical starting point for individual action and program development, as well as a continuing process for keeping activities on track. As we will describe later in this book, a needs assessment can be repeated to monitor program impacts. This process enables our educational and promotional efforts to be guided by a realistic database. Overall, a needs assessment process can assist practitioners in a variety of ways: Program development efforts can be based on reported needs, changes and trends can be assessed over a period of time, individuals and target audiences can be involved in purposeful activities, and the target audience can be more accurately characterized.

What does capacity mean? Capacity refers to both individual and collective resources that can be brought to bear for health enhancement. It includes assets in individuals that can provide certain protective influences affecting whether people engage in certain risk-related behaviors like tobacco use (Atkins, Oman, Vesely, et al., 2002). Clark (2000) has made reference to a matrix of needs and responses that ensures quality of life, referring to individual and collective responses in relation to personal and societal needs. Reference is also made to the importance of developing community capacity and power, which are integral to the enhancement of personal capacity and power needed to ensure quality of life. As Clark (2000) points out, "individuals must develop the perspectives, values, and skills necessary to maintain the quality of their lives as appropriate and desired in their particular community and culture, and they must be enveloped by a society that is socially integrated, is cohesive, and provides moral and material support when needed" (p. 704).

What is a capacity assessment? A capacity assessment is a measure of actual and potential individual, group, and community resources that can be inherent and/or brought to bear for health maintenance and enhancement. From an individual perspective, capacity can be measured in terms of assets or protective factors (Atkins, Oman, Vesely, et al., 2002); at the group or community level, capacity can be considered as unique histories, cultures, structures, personalities, politics, and systems, all brought together for health enhancement (Bond, Glover, Godfrey, et al., 2001; Cheadle, Sullivan, Krieger, et al., 2002). Included in the capacity assessment approach is the community assets mapping process (Parks and Straker, 1996; Kretzmann and McKnight, 1993).

Why conduct a capacity assessment? From a community-based perspective, capacity assessment provides an opportunity to engage multiple stakeholders and others in a review of actual and potential resources that can influence current and future partnership efforts. Capacity assessment also enables individuals to review sources of support in their lives (e.g., individual protective factors, significant others, educational and worksite settings). It is essential to review the actual and potential availability of resources for the sake of establishing realistic project starting points and ascertaining project sustainability.

Balancing Science and Art

Qualitative and Quantitative Issues

Human needs and capacities are diverse and changing. No single approach to assessing them would always be appropriate. Instead, a variety of approaches usually is necessary. One way to expand the approach is to consider the use of both quantitative and qualitative information. Health and human service professionals are familiar with quantitative data. Newspapers are full of statistics describing increases in health care costs, changes in the incidence of specific diseases, and various lifestyle trends. Professional journals rely heavily on quantitative data to report the results of scientific and applied research. Most people usually have a greater familiarity, and perhaps security, with numbers. Our society has been conditioned to focus on something ranked number one, rather than number ten.

However, numbers do not always tell the full story. In fact, they can oversimplify matters. For this reason, they need to be balanced with qualitative data. Narrative information is necessary to elaborate on statistical data and to contribute insights. A narrative format can capture variations and exceptions, and portray the needs and available resources as completely as possible. As has been pointed out by Creswell (2003), the qualitative approach is basically an interpretive process with a reliance on text and image data.

As one example, in a given community there could be a relatively high incidence of teenage deaths, in comparison with state statistics. Recent local statistics regarding the causes of teenage deaths might show that motor vehicle accidents represent the leading cause of death. However, other sources of information could include one's co-workers, representatives from local and state organizations, and key individuals in the community. Discussions with these people might reveal contributing factors that are associated with motor vehicle accidents, such as an awareness of increasing alcohol consumption among teens, observed high speed travel on secondary roads, and a sense of increased stress in the family. This qualitative information yields a more complete picture of teenage deaths, and suggests possible contributing factors for the professional to address.

Intuition's Contributions

Our instincts and feelings count in needs and capacity assessments. In addition to gathering quantitative and qualitative information, these more intuitive responses of health and human service professionals and community members are also important, and should not be ignored. At the core, intuition refers to direct insight that is not initially inferred through facts.

Another, more focused approach to comprehending intuition is based on personality type theory, where intuition is described as one of two key constructs within the psychological realm of perception (i.e., all the ways we become aware of things, people, happenings, or ideas). In this context, intuition focuses on possibilities and what "might be," rather than specifics and "what is," which is more of a sensing perspective (Allen and Brock, 2000; Hirsh and Kummerow, 1997). Further, while the perceiving process of "sensing" means that we are becoming aware of things directly through our five senses, "intuition" means that we are indirectly becoming aware of things through considerations of meanings, relationships, and possibilities. Using our intuition typically means reading between and beyond the lines. Allen and Brock (2000) have used the personality type approach effectively in reviewing the distinctions that occur in health care communications. To become more cognizant of differences, the preferences of both the practitioner and the client/patient are assessed, eventually leading to the development of improved written and interactive communications.

Drawing on this orientation, an early study by Agor (1984) examined the value of intuition for making practical management decisions. He cited examples, as well as data from his own research, that demonstrated how some successful managers made major decisions based on intuition. In some cases, intuition took precedence over conflicting or inadequate information. In a national study involving 1,679 managers, Agor found use of intuition to be more prevalent with those advanced in management rank. Top managers in every sample group tested used intuition in decision making to a greater extent than middle- and lower-level managers. This type of finding has been documented by others as well (Roach, 1986; Reynierse, 1991).

When later studies were conducted at the international level, such clear-cut distinctions did not evolve. For example, using a sample of 3,688 Japanese managers, executives, and CEOs, Reynierse (1995) compared their preference data with 1993 data he had collected on 1,952 American managers and executives. While the data for the American executives revealed increasing intuitive preferences at the higher management levels (as predicted), the Japanese data showed a notable intuitive preference at all management levels. This finding may reflect the decision-making distinction between American and Japanese companies: Japanese decision making is highly participatory, in contrast to American approaches in which the decision making and final authority are detailed through job descriptions and organizational frameworks. Obviously, the findings from one cultural context cannot automatically be applied to others.

In a general sense, however, one's intuition increases with experience. New health and human service professionals may not have a wealth of experience on which to draw. There may be a hesitation in trusting individual feelings about needs and priorities, and a desire to rely more extensively on quantitative data. With increasing experience, however, individual insights take on a greater significance in the planning process.

Assumptions and Assessments

Two types of groups are involved in needs and capacity assessments. One group comprises the professionals directly involved in the planning, coordinating, or facilitating of the assessments. They bring to the process health-related expertise, and often previous assessment experience. The other group consists of the target audience or target group. These individuals bring their expectations and life experiences, which help them identify a range of needs, wants, interests, and capacities. They also should be engaged from the outset so that their contributions can be made during the planning, implementation, and evaluation phases, as appropriate.

When the two groups enter into the assessment processes, individuals in both groups bring some assumptions about the needs and resources at hand. These assumptions are intuitive in nature, influenced by the previous experiences, opinions, feelings, and ideas of each individual. Practitioners develop assumptions based on ongoing interaction with community members and other professionals, examination of demographic data and vital statistics, comprehension of the various political and socioeconomic forces influencing the community, and personal insights, awareness, and experience. Members of the target group draw on their own insights and experiences in making their own assumptions.

If accurate, these assumptions can be very helpful in identifying a starting point. They can help to narrow the focus of a too-broad or too-generalized approach to a needs or capacity assessment. Collective assumptions from practitioners and community representatives can be discussed to help guide the assessment process in the right direction.

However, assumptions are not meant to take the place of assessments. In a sense, they act as precursors to sets of reported needs and resources. It is through the assessment process that these assumptions become more clearly defined and are possibly revised, resulting in some specifically identified needs and capacities.

Once specific needs and capacities have been assessed, it is important for the practitioner to offer a summary of the preliminary results to the community representatives. This approach provides all stakeholders with the opportunity to clarify and acknowledge the extent to which the identified needs and resources accurately reflect those of the involved groups. At that point, practitioners and representatives can reach a joint agreement regarding which needs to address and how best to address them with the resources at hand.

Some Basic Premises

Our overall approach to needs and capacity assessment is based on certain premises. Prior to your review of the individual and group needs and capacity assessment processes in the following chapters, consider these grounding points:

1. *People* are important to needs and capacity assessments. Individuals have the capacity to reflect on their health-related needs and to report these needs. Practitioners also can draw from their education and experience to reflect and report on the health-related needs and capacities of the people with whom they work. Importantly, not only do the assessments provide necessary insights and information, but involvement in their planning and implementation can also contribute to the development of meaningful working relationships.

2. The *needs* that people report are realistic issues to consider, particularly when a trend is apparent. We can view reported needs as one source of information. (We will address other sources in the forthcoming chapters.)

3. A *needs assessment* is an applied process for gathering useful information for individual and group planning purposes. Its basic purpose is not to construct or test a scientific hypothesis, although good research

techniques often are used in data collection and analysis. Throughout the book, you will note the focus on better preparing the practitioner to address key needs and capacity assessment issues that have a high potential for being experienced.

4. *Capacity assessments* can be quite varied because they assess individual and group resources over an array of parameters. They can cover distinct time dimensions (past, present, future), settings (local, state, regional, national, international), and contexts (social, cultural, political, and the like). Importantly, such resources need to be considered in as comprehensive a manner as time, fiscal, and human resources will allow.

5. *Planning and advisory committees* are important to the needs and capacity assessment processes. Often, such committees are established after the needs have been determined and the program is about to be planned. Alternatively, planning and advisory committees made up of practitioners and stakeholders (i.e., those involved in and affected by the issues being addressed) can help to plan and conduct the assessments. A committee can determine which kinds of needs and resources to consider, from whom to gather information, and which strategies to use. Committee members also can assist with data collection and analysis. Involving such committees at this early stage can ensure that the program is based on the perceived needs and the available and potential resources of the intended participants.

6. Needs and capacity assessments are *integral parts of the program planning process*. These assessments represent key steps in planning effective health education and health promotion activities.

Summary

This chapter has addressed the value of an increased focus on needs and capacity assessments, questions regarding their nature, some of the basic principles, and our own premises. Human needs and capacities, while complex, are able to be assessed within the context of target group settings and situations that affect those needs and resources. Practitioners also have a context from which to draw preliminary needs- and capacity-related inferences based on their experiences and impressions. However, these are merely starting points for the professional; they offer clues to possible target group needs and capacities. Practitioners must consider the value of determining the prioritized needs and capacities of groups in a structured, collaborative fashion so that effective health education and health promotion efforts can be continued, adjusted, or newly developed as appropriate.

Online Resources

Visit http://healtheducation.jbpub.com/gilmore for links to these Web sites.

Office of Environmental Health Assessments
This Web site is from the Washington State Department of Health and includes definitions of health assessments and health education.

Alberta Consultative Health Research Network
This Web site describes needs assessments and questions to ask before preparing a needs assessment.

Supercourse: Epidemiology, the Internet, and Global Health
This site is a PowerPoint presentation that describes needs assessments.

Laboratory for Community and Economic Development
This site discusses why assessments should be done, who should be involved, what the steps of an assessment are, and where communities can go for help on conducting a needs assessment.

Ohio State University
This site discusses why and how a needs assessment should be used, what the benefits and challenges are to using one, how to plan, and how to report and use the information retrieved.

References

Agor, W. (1984). *Intuitive Management.* Englewood Cliffs, NJ: Prentice Hall.

Allen, J., and Brock, S. (2000). *Health Care Communication Using Personality Type.* Philadelphia: Routledge Publishing.

American Association for Health Education (AAHE); National Commission for Health Education Credentialing (NCHEC); Society for Public Health Education (SOPHE). (1999). *A Competency-Based Framework for Graduate-Level Health Educators.* Allentown, PA: Authors.

Atkins, L., Oman, R., Vesely, S., Aspy, C., and McLeroy, K. (2002). Adolescent Tobacco Use: The Protective Effects of Developmental Assets. *American Journal of Health Promotion,* 16, 198–205.

Bensky, J., and Hietbrink, R. (1994). Getting Down to Business. *Worksite Health,* 1, 25–28.

Bond, L., Glover, S., Godfrey, C., Butler, H., and Patton, G. (2001). Building Capacity for System-Level Change in Schools: Lessons from the Gatehouse Project. *Health Education and Behavior,* 28, 368–383.

Centers for Disease Control and Prevention (CDC). (September 11, 2002). Community Needs Assessment of Lower Manhattan Residents Following the World Trade Center Attacks—Manhattan, New York City, 2001. *Morbidity and Mortality Weekly Report,* 51, 10–13.

Centers for Disease Control and Prevention (CDC). (2003). *A Public Health Action Plan to Prevent Heart Disease and Stroke*. Atlanta, GA: Author.

Cheadle, A., Sullivan, M., Krieger, J., Ciske, S., Shaw, M., Schier, J., and Eisinger, A. (2002). Using a Participatory Approach to Provide Assistance to Community-Based Organizations: The Seattle Partners Community Research Center. *Health Education and Behavior, 29*, 383–394.

Clark, N. (2000). Understanding Individual and Collective Capacity to Enhance Quality of Life. *Health Education and Behavior, 27*, 699–707.

Creswell, J. (2003). *Research Design: Qualitative, Quantitative, and Mixed Methods Approaches*. Thousand Oaks, CA: Sage Publications.

Daley, W., Karpati, A., and Sheik, M. (2002). Needs Assessment of the Displaced Population Following the August 1999 Earthquake in Turkey. *Disasters, 25*, 67–75.

Galea, S., Ahern, J., and Resnick, H. (2002). Psychological Sequelae of the September 11 Terrorist Attacks in New York City. *New England Journal of Medicine, 346*, 982–987.

Gilmore, G., Olsen, L., and Taub, A. (2001). *Competencies Update Project: Promoting Quality Assurance in Health Education*. Bethesda, MD: Bureau of Health Professions, Health Resources and Services Administration, USDHHS, No. 00-257(P).

Hirsh, S., and Kummerow, J. (1997). *Lifetypes*. New York: Warner Books.

Institute of Medicine (IOM). (2001). *Health and Behavior: The Interplay of Biological, Behavioral, and Social Influences*. Washington, DC: National Academies Press.

Institute of Medicine (IOM). (2003). *Who Will Keep the Public Healthy? Educating Public Health Professionals for the 21st Century*. Washington, DC: National Academies Press.

Israel, B., Lichtenstein, R., Lantz, P., McGranaghan, R., Allen, A., Guzman, J., Softley, D., and Maciak, B. (2001). The Detroit Community Academic Urban Research Center: Development, Implementation, and Evaluation. *Journal of Public Health Management and Practice, 7*, 1–19.

Kretzmann, J., and McKnight, J. (1993). *Building Communities from the Inside Out*. Chicago: ACTA Publications.

Miller, R., Bedney, B., and Guenther-Grey, C. (2003). Assessing Organizational Capacity to Deliver HIV Prevention Services Collaboratively: Tales from the Field. *Health Education and Behavior, 30*, 582–600.

National Commission for Health Education Credentialing (NCHEC). (1996). *A Competency-Based Framework for Professional Development of Certified Health Education Specialists*. Allentown, PA: Author.

Office of Disease Prevention and Health Promotion. (2001). *Healthy People in Healthy Communities: A Community Planning Guide Using Healthy People 2010*. Rockville, MD: Office of Public Health and Science, U.S. Public Health Service.

Oldenburg, B., Sallis, J., Harris, D., and Owen, N. (2002). Checklist of Health Promotion Environments at Worksites (CHEW): Development and Measurement Characteristics. *American Journal of Health Promotion, 16*, 288–299.

Parks, C., and Straker, H. (1996). Community Assets Mapping: Community Health Assessment with a Different Twist. *Journal of Health Education, 27,* 321–323.

Pratt, M., McDonald, S., Libby, P., Oberle, M., and Liang, A. (1996). Local Health Departments in Washington State Use APEX to Assess Capacity. *Public Health Reports,* 111, 87–91.

Reynierse, J. (1995). A Comparative Analysis of Japanese and American Management Types Through Organizational Levels in Business and Industry. *Journal of Psychological Type, 33,* 19–32.

Reynierse, J. (1991). The Psychological Types of Outplaced Executives. *Journal of Psychological Type, 25,* 11–23.

Roach, B. (1986). Organizational Decision-Makers: Different Types for Different Levels. *Journal of Psychological Type, 12,* 16–24.

Schulz, A., Krieger, J., and Galea, S. (2002). Addressing Social Determinants of Health: Community-Based Participatory Approaches to Research and Practice. *Health Education and Behavior, 29,* 287–295.

Taintor, Z. (2003). Addressing Mental Health Needs. In B. Levy & V. Sidel (Eds.), *Terrorism and Public Health: A Balanced Approach to Strengthening Systems and Protecting People* (pp. 49–68). New York: Oxford University Press.

U.S. Department of Health and Human Services (USDHHS). (2000). *Healthy People 2010: Understanding and Improving Health.* Washington, DC: U.S. Government Printing Office.

Needs and Capacity Assessments within the Bigger Picture

Introduction

Needs and capacity assessments for health education and health promotion do not stand alone. Rather, they are part of a bigger picture—namely, the development, implementation, and evaluation of health education strategies for health promotional purposes. This chapter reviews key contexts for the assessment strategies detailed in later chapters. These include the meanings of health as related to health promotion and health education; how needs and capacity assessments fit into program development; the roles of advisory groups, planning committees, and community coalitions; key data collection considerations; and needs prioritization.

The Context of Health, Health Promotion, and Health Education

The terms "health promotion" and "health education" encompass broad dimensions in addressing *health*, a term which also has a variety of definitions. The World Health Organization's (WHO) definition of health in 1948 moved us from a static, singular depiction of one's physical status into a more multidimensional perspective of "a state of complete physical, mental and social well-being—not merely the absence of disease, or infirmity" (USDHHS, November 2000, p. 4; World Health Organization, 1985). In the past, that definition has been critiqued by some as more of an ideal than a reality that can feasibly be obtained. In 1987, Noack offered a definition of health that was more process and systems oriented, and more of an operational definition of health: "a state of dynamic balance—or more appropriately as a process maintaining such a state—within any given subsystem, such as an organ, an individual, a social group, or a community" (p. 14). He added that health has two key dimensions: health balance (a dynamic equilibrium) and health potential (capacity for balance between person and environment), at the individual and community levels in both instances. Examples of health balance at the individual and community levels would be a relaxed state and a sense of family well-being in the community, respectively. Examples of health potential at the same levels would be nutritional status and the proportion of a health agency's budget aligned with health promotion activities, respectively.

While the WHO perspective is considered to offer a broad definition of health, others have taken a more narrow approach to the measurement of health in the United States by focusing on ill health in its severe manifestations as diagnosed through clinical tests (USDHHS, November 2000). As pointed out by the CDC, other important aspects of individual or community health, such as disease-related dysfunction and disability, injuries, and other health problems, may be missed in taking such a measurement. The public health community currently views health status as a multidimensional construct, which includes "premature mortality and life expectancy, various symptoms and physiologic states, physical functions, emotional and cognitive functions, and perceptions about present and future health" (USDHHS, November 2000, p. 5). Taking such a perspective of health moves it into the realm of quality of life, which refers to "an overall sense of well-being, including aspects of happiness and satisfaction with life as a whole" (USDHHS, November 2000, p. 5). In addition to health, other domains are embodied within quality of life—for example, jobs, housing, schools, and one's neighborhood.

More recently, a new metric has emerged from this more inclusive perspective: health-related quality of life (HRQOL). It includes "those aspects of overall quality of life that can be clearly shown to affect health—either physical or mental" (USDHHS, November 2000, p. 6). Numerous reports are using this measurement approach to quantify HRQOL in a variety of public health issues (USDHHS, January 2001; USDHHS, May 2000; USDHHS, April 2000; Campbell, Crews, Moriarty, et al., 1999; Hennessy, Moriarty, Zack, et al., 1994).

Contributing to this broader approach, the Institute of Medicine's 2001 report, *Health and Behavior: The Interplay of Biological, Behavioral, and Social Influences,* views health from a perspective in which any health problems fall along a continuum based on the influence of various risk factors that can range from bio-behavioral (e.g., stress response, coping patterns), to behavioral (e.g., tobacco use, diet, physical activity), to social (e.g., positive relationship pathways, social networking, socioeconomic status) (Pellmar, Brandt, and Baird, 2002). Additionally, interactions among risk factors can influence health (Mokdad et al., 2004). These interactions particularly become apparent in the realm of socioeconomic factors. For instance, among the socioeconomically advantaged, lower mortality, morbidity, and disability rates have been observed over time. Individuals who are poor are more likely to engage in risk-related behaviors and are less likely to engage in health-promotional behaviors (Pellmar, Brandt, and Baird, 2002). As has been pointed out by Green (1999), "a balanced portfolio of factors under greater control of individuals and more distal risk conditions controlled by others, as determinants of health, is needed to correct the poor penetration by health programs in poor and marginalized populations" (p. 81). Importantly, key reports and frameworks for the twenty-first century are being grounded in the more comprehensive approach to health impacts offered by our better understanding of the determinants of health (Mokdad et al., 2004; Committee on Assuring the Health of the Public in the 21st Century, 2003; Gebbie, Rosenstock, and Hernandez, 2003). Gebbie and colleagues (2003) have emphasized that practitioners "must be aware of not only the biological risk factors affecting health; they must also understand the environmental, social, and behavioral contexts within which individuals and populations operate in order to identify factors that may hinder or promote the success of their interventions" (p. 34).

As emphasized by Cromley and McLafferty (2002), an essential consideration for our understanding of health is the person within an environmental context that is "connected to natural, social, and economic processes that operate on the local, regional, and global scales" (p. 2). They note that not all factors affecting our state of health are under our control, because "how people behave contributes to their health status, but we cannot divorce behavior from the environmental and social contexts in which it occurs" (p. 2).

The Committee on Assuring the Health of the Public in the 21st Century (2003), in reviewing the major trends influencing the health of the United States, cited three in particular:

1. Population growth and demographic change, with the "population growing larger, older, and more racially and ethnically diverse, with a higher incidence of chronic disease;
2. Technical and scientific advances, which "create new channels for information and communication, as well as novel ways of preventing and treating disease; and
3. Globalization and health, to include the "geopolitical and economic challenge of globalization, including international terrorism" (pp. 34–41).

These contexts are viewed as both opportunities and threats.

Clearly, defining health involves numerous dimensions that are not easily quantifiable. This complexity heightens even further as we advance into a more specific review into the contexts of health promotion and health education.

Health promotion can be viewed as a collective effort in health enhancement. The process has been defined by the Joint Committee on Health Education and Promotion Terminology as "any planned combination of educational, political, environmental, regulatory, or organizational mechanisms that supports actions and conditions of living conducive to the health of individuals, groups, and communities" (2001, p. 101). This definition expands upon the definition offered by Green and Kreuter (1999) by including the environmental dimension. Importantly, Breslow (1999) refers to health promotion as a "more recent and elusive concept that has appeared prominently in the health lexicon only during the latter part of the 20th century" (p. 1030). He differentiates health promotion from disease prevention in that the former "means facilitating at least the maintenance of a person's current position on the continuum (degree of health) and, ideally, advancing toward its positive end (health). Disease prevention, on the other hand, means avoiding specific diseases that carry one toward the negative end (infirmity)" (p. 1032). Additionally, he calls for not only a maintenance of balance in one's life, but also attempts to maximize one's enjoyment potential. From more of a global perspective, health promotion was defined by the WHO's Working Group on Concepts and Principles of Health Promotion (1987, p. 654) as the process of enabling people to increase control over, and to improve, their health. This promotional perspective is derived from a conception of health as the extent to which an individual or group is able to realize aspirations and satisfy needs, and to change or cope with the environment. Health in this context is seen as a "resource of everyday life, not the objective of living; it is a positive concept emphasizing social and personal resources as well as physical capacities." Basic characteristics of health promotion cited by the Working Group on Concepts and Principles (1987, p. 654) were the following:

1. Enabling people to take control over, and responsibility for, their health as an important component of everyday life—both as spontaneous and as organized action for health
2. Requiring the close cooperation of sectors beyond the health services, reflecting the diversity of conditions that influence health
3. Combining diverse, but complementary, methods or approaches, including communication, education, legislation, fiscal measures, organizational changes, community development, and spontaneous local activities against health hazards
4. Encouraging effective and concrete public participation encompassing the development of individual and collective problem-solving and decision-making skills, and involving health professionals in education and health advocacy, particularly those in primary care

In attempting to achieve these aspects of health promotion, recommendations were advanced that focused on equitable health policies, work and home environments conducive to health, establishment of social networks, social support, coping strategies, and health-related lifestyles. Additionally, there was a call for increases in knowledge as drawn from epidemiology, social, and other sciences. With this as background, the Working Group on Concepts and Principles (1987, p. 657) cited a series of selected considerations for prioritizing health promotion policy development:

- Indicators of health and their population distributions
- Current population knowledge, skills, and health practices
- Current policies in government and other sectors
- Expected impact on health
- Economic constraints and benefits
- Social and cultural acceptability
- Political feasibility

In reviewing health promotion in a community context, Green and Raeburn (1990) refer to its major purpose being the "increasing transfer of control of important resources in health, notably knowledge, skills, authority, and money, to the community" (p. 37). They expand on this perspective by calling for an enabling approach in which the people of a community establish their own activities for improved health in accordance with their understanding of needs. In addition to the potential health benefits for the community using this self-help approach, there are the benefits of an increased sense of social support from peers and a sense of control in their own lives. Pellmar et al. (2002) refer to several lessons learned from community intervention experiences as including the importance of the community itself in defining needs and priorities, rather than an outside organizer, and the need for community diagnosis and assessment to be conducted in an ongoing manner.

Health education is an educational context within health promotion. Although numerous definitions of health education exist, we have found that much of what is practiced relates to the blending of two widely recognized definitions. The Joint Committee on Health Education and Promotion Terminology (2001) defines health education as "any combination of planned learning experiences based on sound theories that provide individuals, groups, and communities the opportunity to acquire information and the skills needed to make quality health decisions" (p. 99). Notably, the theoretical basis for the learning, coupled with information and skills acquisition for health-related decision making, represent key ingredients. Green and Kreuter (1999) define health education as "any combination of learning experiences designed to predispose, enable, and reinforce voluntary behavior conducive to health in individuals, groups, or communities" (p. 506). In doing so, they incorporate the three key factors having the potential to influence voluntary health behavior: predisposing factors, which "include a person or population's knowledge, attitudes, beliefs, values, and perceptions that facilitate or hinder motivation for change"; enabling factors, which "are those skills, resources, or barriers that can help or hinder the desired behavioral changes as well as environmental changes"; and reinforcing factors, which are "the rewards received and the feedback the learner receives from others following adoption of a behavior" (pp. 40–41). We believe a blending of these two seminal definitions can best guide the health educator's efforts. The view of the health educator as planning educational experiences guided by theory that voluntarily foster health enhancement is a key grounding point in this book.

How Needs and Capacity Assessments Fit into Program Planning

Many distinctive approaches to health education planning are utilized, usually focusing on many or all of the generic phases of assessing needs, stating the issues or problems to be addressed, developing goals and objectives, reviewing resources (capacities) and barriers, determining methods, implementing, and evaluating. A specific example includes the PRECEDE-PROCEED approach (Green and Kreuter, 1999), which emphasizes problem-aligned deductive diagnoses. The process comprises the phases depicted in **Figure 1**.

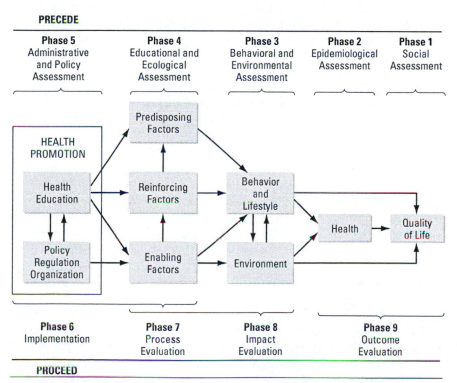

FIGURE 1

Generic representation of the PRECEDE-PROCEED model as advanced by Lawrence Green and Marshall Kreuter. From: Green, L. and Kreuter, M. (1999). *Health Promotion Planning: An Educational and Ecological Approach.* Mountain View, California: Mayfield Publishing Company. Reproduced with the permission of The McGraw-Hill Companies.

PRECEDE is an acronym for Predisposing, Reinforcing, and Enabling Constructs in Educational/ecological Diagnosis and Evaluation, with the goal of assuring comprehensive *assessment* and *planning* phases. Working in tandem with these phases is the PROCEED approach, which is an acronym for Policy, Regulatory, and Organizational Constructs in Educational and Environmental Development; here the goal is to address the *implementation* and *evaluation* components of health education and health promotion endeavors. As Green and Kreuter (1999) have pointed out, "the identification of priorities in one phase of PRECEDE leads to quantitative objectives that become goals and targets in the implementation phase of PROCEED. They then become the standards of acceptability or criteria of success in the evaluation phases of PROCEED" (p. 34). Needs and capacity assessments are particularly aligned with the PRECEDE portion of the model (Green and Kreuter, 1999, pp. 32–43, 188–217). Phases 1–4 of PRECEDE address individual and group needs through the social, epidemiological, behavioral, environmental, educational, and ecological *needs assessments*. Phase 5 addresses the administrative and policy assessments related to organizational and community *capacity* (e.g., the resources and policies in place).

Given the wide acceptance of the PRECEDE-PROCEED model for health promotion planning, we believe there is value for the professional to give strong consideration to its utility in program development. Green and Kreuter (1999) emphasize that it is not to be considered the only approach for health promotional efforts, but it does appropriately address both health promotion and health education through a comprehensive planning approach. We believe that the model is one of the more complete planning approaches because of this comprehensive focus.

More recently, Green and Kreuter (personal correspondence with Lawrence Green, June 17 and September 19, 2003) have been in the process of enhancing their model. For example, their fourth edition (2005) merges the epidemiological, behavioral, and environmental assessment phases (to include genetics) into one phase. Realizing that individuals become engaged with the model at different phases of their professional activities, an algorithm is provided to recognize their previous project endeavors as they connect with different points in the model. Green and Kreuter are moving in this direction to enable professionals to focus on those phases that will have value to them depending on the project stage in which they are currently engaged. To their credit, Green and Kreuter's revision is based to a large extent on the continuing feedback they seek from the field to assure that their model remains practical and up-to-date. Current information and endnote updates regarding the PRECEDE-PROCEED model can be accessed through their Web site: http://www.lgreen.net.

Another helpful planning perspective offered as an outgrowth of the national health initiative, *Healthy People 2010: Healthy People in Healthy Communities,* is entitled *MAP-IT* (USDHHS, February 2001). This easy-to-use format is aligned with the two major goals of (1) increasing the quality of years of healthy life and (2) eliminating health disparities. While *healthy life* refers to both qualitative and quantitative dimensions as described earlier in Chapter 1 (USDHHS, January 2000), *health disparities* is defined as the "differences in the burden and impact of disease among different populations, defined, for example, by sex, race or ethnicity, education or income, disability, place of residence, or sexual orientation" (USDHHS, 2003, p. A-3). Coupled with the two overarching goals are ten priorities (10 Leading Health Indicators): physical activity; overweight and obesity; tobacco use; substance abuse; responsible sexual behavior; mental health; injury and violence; environmental quality; immunization; and access to health care. Within the context of these key elements in the national framework for health enhancement, the *MAP-IT* model provides the following actions:

- Mobilize individuals and organizations that care about the health of your community into a coalition
- Assess the areas of greatest need in your community as well as the resources and other strengths that you can tap into to address those areas
- Plan your approach—start with a vision of where you want to be as a community, and then add strategies and action steps to help you achieve that vision
- Implement your plan using concrete action steps that can be monitored and will make a difference
- Track your progress over time (p. 7)

Mobilizing refers to the development of a community coalition, as appropriate, by bringing together committed individuals and organizations gathered around a vision of how the coalition would like the community to be.

Assessing refers to the process of determining the health issues of greatest importance in the community and ascertaining the available strengths and resources. Both primary and secondary data should be compiled into baseline information prior to the initiation of any action or program.

Planning includes the development of objectives that have specific targets for change (criteria) in comparison to the baseline data; action steps, which are concrete actions in alignment with the objectives; assigned responsibilities to facilitate the action plan; and a proposed timeline.

Implementing involves taking the concrete actions specified in the action plan, along with monitoring the events as they transpire.

Tracking entails a two-part evaluation phase including progress reviews and the assurance of continuing support. As a part of this phase, the recommendation is made to celebrate small successes en route to the larger goal (overall direction).

Within the context of planning for worksite health promotion, Bensky and Hietbrink (1994) have suggested starting with an STP team, which focuses on the current Situation, the Target outcome for health promotional activity, and the proposed Plan. This team is then guided by considerations of issues that influence the decisions to be made, information that will clarify any assumptions about the issues, interpretation of what the information means, implications about how the program will be affected if the interpretation is accurate, and initiative regarding which actions to take. Bensky and Hietbrink's (1994) rather straightforward planning framework addresses the following points: (1) assessment of the situation from a who, what, when, where, and why perspective (this incorporates a SWOT analysis, which reviews any current program Strengths and Weaknesses, as well as Opportunities and Threats to programming in the next year); (2) setting the goals; (3) developing appropriate strategies; and (4) writing a plan that can achieve buy-in by those most directly affected by the initiative.

There is no shortage of quality planning approaches available with which to expand on traditional and nontraditional planning models. The reader is encouraged to review texts that take a more health promotional perspective (i.e., overall health enhancement), such as McKenzie and Smeltzer (1997) and Timmreck (2003). The generic planning model described by McKenzie and Smeltzer (1997) can be a helpful starting point for the practitioner. This more traditional approach to planning offers the following components:

- Assessing *needs*
- Identifying *problems*
- Developing *goals* and *objectives*
- Creating *interventions*
- *Implementing* the intervention
- *Evaluating* the results

Initially, it will be helpful to the practitioner to track these procedures by using the highlighted entities as prompts while health education and health promotion strategies are being developed. Other aspects of planning, such as assessing the capacity of an organization or community to support change, eventually will need to be taken into consideration as well. Readers who have aligned themselves successfully with a particular health education planning process are advised to continue with that approach. The needs and capacity assessment strategies described in this book will provide a starting point for issue and resource identification for a wide array of planning models.

Capacity-Focused Assessments

As pointed out earlier, capacity assessments can be included in other planning models under different names (e.g., the Administrative and Policy assessment in the PRECEDE-PROCEED model). Importantly, capacity assessments can be conducted at the organizational and community-based levels to assess actual and potential resources, policies, and support entities that will fortify and sustain project and program endeavors. As pointed out by Bartholomew, Parcel, Kok, and Gottlieb (2001), at the outset of program planning, assessing community-based competencies and resources focuses attention on the importance of capacity enhancement during the development and implementation phases of planning.

Along these lines, Kretzmann and McKnight (1993) pioneered capacity-focused, or asset-based, approaches to community planning. The driving force behind this approach initially was the focus on rebuilding troubled communities by undertaking asset-based community development, rather than by focusing on the needs, deficiencies, and problems of a community. The latter approach is believed to foster client neighborhoods in which there is little or no empowerment for the residents due to reliance on outside experts, fragmented attempts at solutions that focus on isolated clients rather than the community as a whole, funding that is basically directed toward service providers, and consequently a deepening sense of dependence and hopelessness among the residents. As an alternative, capacity-focused community development seeks to build on the "capacities, skills, and assets of lower income people and their neighborhoods" (Kretzmann and McKnight, 1993, p. 5). The assets are established based on the assessment of contributions that can be made by individuals, citizens' associations (e.g., churches, cultural groups), and local institutions (e.g., businesses, schools, libraries, health care facilities). This approach is designed to foster an internal focus for problem solving and relationship building that emphasizes "the primacy of local definition, investment, creativity, hope and control" (Kretzmann and McKnight, 1993, p. 9).

The primary capacity-focused assessment process advanced by Kretzmann and McKnight (1993), known as the Capacity Inventory, comprises four parts seeking the following information: skills learned at home, in the community, or in the workplace; experience in community activities and future participation possibilities; business interests and experiences; and personal information. For the most part, this assessment has been implemented as a face-to-face interview, but it can also be modified for use as a survey instrument that individuals complete on their own. The Capacity Inventory is designed to assess how a particular individual can contribute to the community development process. An array of helpful capacity inventory examples are provided in workbooks by Kretzmann, McKnight, and Puntenney (1998), Kretzmann, McKnight, and Sheehan (1997), and Dewar (1997).

Using today's technology, the results of such capacity and needs assessments can be plotted using printed maps as well as geographic information systems (GIS), which are computer-based systems for integrating and analyzing geographic information, thereby enabling spatial relationships between objects to be displayed (e.g., concentrations of certain community-based services in selected census tracks). The convenience and timeliness of a GIS approach facilitates the development of "databases of health events located on the earth's surface that can be processed and stored by computers, keeping track of changes by adding and deleting events from those databases, and editing the location and public health attributes of these events" (Cromley and McLafferty, 2002, p. 19).

The use of a capacity-based approach to assessment and information plotting aligns with the focus on the empowerment of the community to be involved in actions for improvement. This view of empowerment has been defined by Wallerstein (1992) as "a social-action process that promotes participation of people, organizations, and communities towards the goals of increased individual and community control, political efficacy, improved quality of community life, and social justice" (p. 198). From this perspective, community empowerment could potentially address the effects of powerlessness (lack of control, which is considered to be a broad risk factor for disease).

These perspectives serve to expand one's understanding of health issues and potential directions for health enhancement. As summarized by Robertson and Minkler (1994), prominent features of such a perspective include the following:

1. Broadening the definition of health and its determination to include the social and economic context within which health—or, more precisely, nonhealth—is produced
2. Going beyond the earlier emphasis on individual lifestyle strategies to apply health to broader social and political strategies
3. Embracing the concept of empowerment—individual and collective— as a key health promotion strategy
4. Advocating the participation of the community in identifying health problems and strategies for addressing those problems (p. 296)

Within this context, Robertson and Minkler (1994) caution that communities are not homogeneous, so many diverse areas of interest may exist. It is possible that conflict, rather than consensus, can be generated when using a community-driven process, where "communities may assess social problems and propose solutions that reflect racism, sexism, ageism, or other problematic and divisive approaches" (p. 307).

With these cautions and considerations in mind, we view the capacity-focused approach to resource, policy, and support entity assessment as complementing needs assessment activities and as aligning with the planning models described previously. Another planning approach in which both needs and capacity assessments are undertaken is through the application of the logic model.

Logic Models

The logic model approach (also termed the "model of change" or "causal chain" approach) to program planning enables the professional to link program inputs and activities to program outcomes. The process also can be of value in generating planner and stakeholder buy-in through a concise review of how the program design will make a difference for program participants and the overall community (Harvard Family Research Project, 2002). **Figure 2** depicts basic logic model considerations (MacDonald, Starr, Schooley, et al., 2001).

Usually initiated following the assessment of needs, the *inputs* phase encompasses the assessment of capacity, which can include direct and in-kind funding, staffing, partner organizations, equipment, and materials. *Activities* are the events that take place as a part of the program, such as developing a media plan and forming coalitions. *Outputs* are the direct products of the activities of the program, such as a written plan for a population-specific media plan and quantification of the actions taken (e.g., the number of smokers enrolled in a cessation program). *Outcomes* refer to the intended program effects (expected changes). *Short-term* outcomes entail the immediate effects on the target audience, usually in terms of knowledge, attitudes, and skills (e.g., a more positive attitude toward smoke-free policies among business owners). *Intermediate* outcomes refer primarily to behavior and policy changes (e.g., an increase in the percentage of adults who implement household smoking restrictions, and the adoption of clean indoor-air policies). *Long-term* outcomes are changes that occur over much longer periods of time, such as years (e.g., decreases in the prevalence of tobacco use, and reduced tobacco-related morbidity and mortality among the target populations.) Logic model development moves from right to left. A detailed example of a smoking cessation promotion effort for youth and adults is presented in **Figure 3**.

Advisory and Planning Committees

One very helpful method to develop a clearer and more comprehensive planning approach is to establish a committee. Two types of committees can be organized: advisory and planning committees. An **advisory committee** usually consists of individuals who are in a position to periodically report on their actual experiences related to some common issue. Members of this committee are then able to offer their advice to a key individual who is bringing them together, or to another group that will be making programmatic decisions. A **planning committee** may be made up of advisory committee members, experts, and agency staff. Its life span may be episodic (with limited duration) or continuing (ongoing). In some instances advisory committees have been

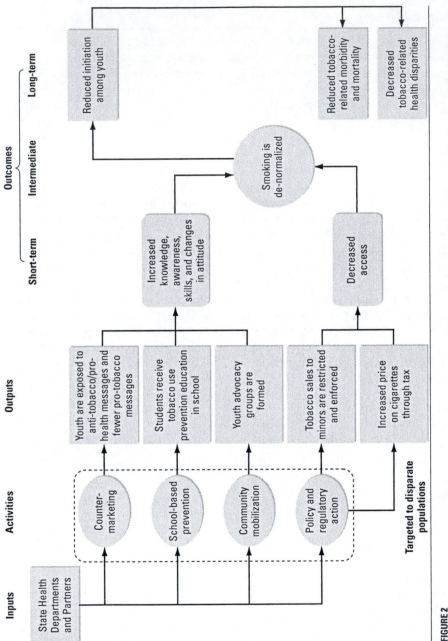

FIGURE 2

Logic model for preventing the initiation of tobacco use among young people. From: MacDonald, G., Starr, G., Schooley, M., Yee, S., Klimowski, K., and Turner, K. (2001). *Introduction to Program Evaluation for Comprehensive Tobacco Control Programs.* Atlanta: Centers for Disease Control and Prevention, Office on Smoking and Health.

28

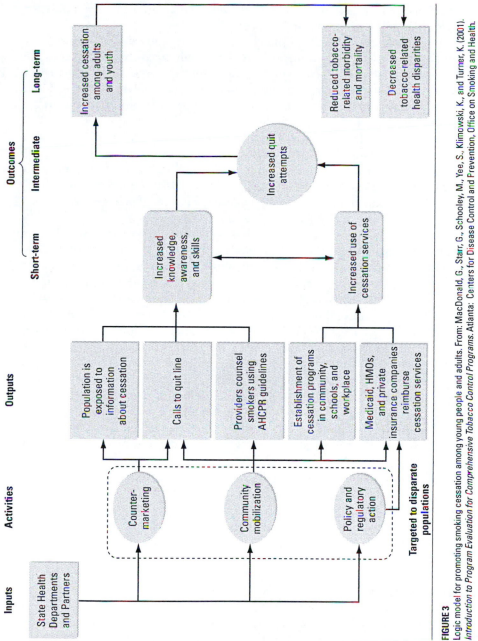

FIGURE 3

Logic model for promoting smoking cessation among young people and adults. From: MacDonald, G., Starr, G., Schooley, M., Yee, S., Klimowski, K., and Turner, K. (2001). *Introduction to Program Evaluation for Comprehensive Tobacco Control Programs.* Atlanta: Centers for Disease Control and Prevention, Office on Smoking and Health.

transformed into planning committees, with the addition of key people, so that a particular program can be developed.

Both types of committees usually share one common denominator: They are task oriented. In addition, both types of committees are important to the long-term assessment processes. They enable firsthand insights and experiences to be offered, they encourage brainstorming, and, particularly in the planning committee process, their members can make an early commitment to undertake key program planning responsibilities at appropriate times.

McKenzie and Smeltzer (1997) have cited a helpful series of guidelines for setting up a committee. An overriding consideration is the selection of individuals from a variety of groups, to include all segments of the program's target populations, along with other stakeholders (those having something to lose or to gain in the process). Engendering a feeling of program ownership is considered to be a key aspect of the committee process.

One can find many examples of advisory and planning groups that have a needs and capacity assessment responsibility. For instance, in the city of Penrith, Australia, a ten-year project focusing on improving a community's food system so as to enhance overall nutrition status is guided by a Food Policy Committee. The committee consists of city councilors as well as representatives from public health and agricultural departments, health-related university departments, food processing and grocery retailing, banking, and the chamber of commerce, among others. The committee operates with a rather high degree of formality guided by a multiyear strategic plan. Included in the committee's numerous responsibilities are the assessment of needs, capacities, opportunities, and relationship development for the furtherance of improved nutritional practices. It has not been an easy task for either the committee or other partners in the project. As Webb et al. (2001) point out, "the challenge remains to document the impact of the project on the local food system and on the capacity of community organizations to reform and implement food policies consistent with improved nutrition" (p. 317). Importantly, this type of committee structure has fostered the institutionalization of the project into the activities of local government.

As another example, a Community Advisory Board was established as part of a community-wide campaign to reduce the cigarette smoking levels in a predominantly African American community in Richmond, California (Hunkeler, Davis, McNeil, et al., 1990). The effort was based on the assumption that "changing the health norms and beliefs of an entire community will change the health habits of individuals" (p. 278). The 30-member board met monthly for three years, advising the campaign workers on almost every aspect of the project. Of interest, rather than setting up ongoing task forces, board members chose instead to establish small working groups with specific assignments addressed through one or two meetings. Organizers believed that the incorporation of the Community Advisory Board legitimized the effort and assured community ownership.

Community-Based Coalitions

On a larger planning scale, community coalitions can be formed as inter-organizational and cooperative groups that establish formal, multipurpose, and long-term alliances (Butterfoss, Goodman, and Wandersman, 1993). The following characteristics more fully describe the uniqueness of coalitions and their purposes:

1. Coalitions enable organizations to become involved in new and broader issues without assuming the sole responsibility for managing or developing those issues.
2. Coalitions can demonstrate and develop widespread public support for issues, actions, or unmet needs.
3. Coalitions can maximize the power of individuals and groups through joint action.
4. Coalitions can minimize the duplication of effort and services.
5. Coalitions can help mobilize more talents, resources, and approaches to influence an issue than any single organization could achieve alone.
6. Coalitions can provide an avenue for recruiting participants from diverse constituencies, such as political, business, human service, social, and religious groups, as well as less organized grassroots groups and individuals.
7. The flexible nature of coalitions allows them to exploit new resources in changing situations (Butterfoss, Goodman, and Wandersman, 1993, p. 315).

Florin, Mitchell, and Stevenson (1993) detail seven stages of coalition development:

1. Initial mobilization, which involves participant recruitment and community constituency engagement
2. Establishing an organizational structure for the working group
3. Building a capacity for action, which involves member skills development and networking
4. Planning for action, which includes the assessment of perceived needs of community constituencies, goal and objective setting, and planning intervention strategies
5. Implementing activities based on a sequential work plan
6. Refining the program based upon evaluation data
7. Institutionalizing the membership process and organizational buy-in

These authors have described the activities of 35 community coalitions that were organized to address alcohol and other drug abuse prevention, particularly from the perspective of their training and technical assistance needs. Among the various needs assessments employed by the coalitions, they noted the use of surveys, focus groups, and town meetings. Plans of action were developed from the assessment data. The relationship between the assessments and the resulting plans could not be evaluated, however, because insufficient information regarding the needs assessment processes was provided in the plans. Overall, the coalition process facilitates collaborative efforts in addressing health-related issues in the community. Due to the usual large-scale nature of a coalition, as well as the ability of organizations to freely enter or leave the structure, considerable effort needs to be directed toward the establishment of committed leadership and interorganizational communication (Bracht and Gleason, 1990).

Data Collection Considerations

Key Informant Insights

Additional insights can be gained from contact with individuals, or **key informants**, who are able to express their perceptions of the needs of others. Such individuals can include community leaders, health and human service professionals, leaders of religious organizations, public officials, educators, and the like. Many times, the information and insights provided by these sources can help to frame key areas of need, which then can be followed up through more definitive needs assessment strategies.

Such a process was employed by one of the authors (GDG) in his needs and capacity assessment work in Dubna, Russia (Gilmore and Hartigan, 1998). Key questions were developed for use during each interview session with health and human service professionals in that city. The overall focus of the assessment and questions had to do with key health-related risk and protective factors affecting the public in Dubna. The key informant information provided a basis for more involved follow-up assessments (e.g., questionnaire and group interviews), eventually leading to a city-wide program development and evaluation. The key informant information assisted the project staff in properly delimiting the objectives and educational methods eventually employed.

Bond et al. (2001), as part of their Gateway Project, incorporated several data-gathering approaches in their mental health promotion capacity assessments in secondary schools, including key informant interviews. The key informants were individuals who held various coordinating positions in the intervention schools, such as assistant principals, curriculum coordinators, and student welfare coordinators. The resulting key informant insights were then combined with other sources of information, such as field notes, surveys, background audits, and student and teacher assessments. Bond et al.'s report specifies how this multiyear project has resulted in system-level changes (e.g., through networks of support and school-based health enhancement teams) based on their capacity-building endeavors.

The process of interviewing key informants is discussed further in Chapter 5.

Secondary Information

As practitioners, we gain insights from a variety of sources. In Chapter 1, we referred to insights as being derived from experience and intuition—understandings that have arisen through our collective professional involvement in health-related matters, rather than as specific results of preplanned assessments. These insights are important in our work and form a backdrop against which we can analyze the findings of our intentional assessment efforts. In a more structured fashion, additional background and supplemental information can be garnered through a review of **secondary information,** which offers social and health indicators for inferential purposes.

Important insights can be derived from analyzing raw data and published data summaries. These data are termed secondary information sources because the analyst did not collect and compile the original data. Sources of these data compilations include libraries, reports of experts and authorities, agency and organizational reports, and commercial information services. Compiled health-related information abounds, as exemplified by reports from the U.S. Census, *Morbidity and Mortality Weekly Report* (MMWR) from the Massachusetts Medical Society, and the *Monthly Vital Statistics Report* (MVSR) from the National Center for Health Statistics (NCHS) at the Centers for Disease Control and Prevention (CDC).

Secondary information can be derived from local, state, national, and international sources. It can be obtained directly from the publisher (in many instances free of charge and in an ongoing manner from public agencies) or indirectly through a library. In some instances, specific documents will be on hand or easily obtainable. In other circumstances, one will have a general idea about the type of information required, but will not be able to cite a specific reference. In these cases, guides and directories are most beneficial.

Examples of data sources at the local level include those maintained by a vital statistics section of a local health department, economic and human resource information available from a human services office, and regional health-related data collected by a health planning agency. Particularly in more rural settings, helpful morbidity and mortality insights can be gained through hospital and coroner records.

At the national level, valuable data and informational updates are provided by the MMWR, MVSR, and NCHS reports, as well as the *Guide to Federal Statistics, A Selected List,* published by the Bureau of the U.S. Census, and *Guide to U.S. Government Statistics*. The National Center for Health Statistics (NCHS) provides important U.S. trend data over time, such as the 1960–2000 overweight and obesity data for adults and youths (see **Figure 4**). Distinct, consistent increases over the years in both overweight and obesity levels signal the high-priority need for key lifestyle-change intervention strategies. Additional resources include the *Statistical Abstract of the United States* and special reports incorporating data from Standard Metropolitan Statistical Areas (SMSAs), with each SMSA being a single county or cluster of contiguous

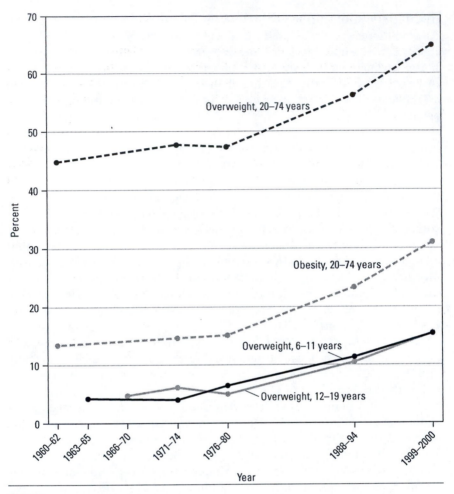

FIGURE 4

Overweight and obesity by age, United States, 1960–2000.

NOTES: Percents for adults are age-adjusted.

Overweight for children is defined as a body mass index (BMI) at or above the sex- and age-specific 95th percentile BMI cut points from the 2000 CDC Growth Charts: United States. Overweight for adults is defined as a BMI greater than or equal to 25 and obesity as a BMI greater than or equal to 30. Obesity is a subset of the percent with overweight. See Data Table for data points graphed, standard errors, and additional notes.

SOURCES: Centers for Disease Control and Prevention, National Center for Health Statistics, National Health Examination Survey, and National Health and Nutrition Examination Survey.

counties that has at least one city with a minimum of 50,000 people. A comprehensive overview of sources of electronic and print-related surveillance systems is provided in Teutsch and Churchill (2000). Of note, this source provides a comprehensive review of measures and determinants (direct, indirect, remote, and underlying) of health status, in addition to addressing the strategies and capacities for health improvement (see Parrish and McDonnell, 2000).

Highly regarded international resources include those provided by the World Health Organization, such as *World Health Statistics* and *Weekly Epidemiological Record*. An overview of available international data sources is provided by the *Directory of United Nations Information Systems and Services.*

These types of sources provide health-related statistical data. Additionally, one can examine demographic data on population patterns, absenteeism records for work and school, income distribution, and political preferences. When we examine this broader context of statistical and demographic data across a population, we are reviewing **social indicators** (see Shi, 1997; Doyle and Ward, 2001). These data can be subjective or objective, direct (data with direct implications, such as achievement test scores) or indirect measures (data used to proxy possible effects, such as the number in a given school receiving AFDC assistance), or descriptive (descriptions of social characteristics) or analytic (relationships among characteristics). Examination of such social indicators can provide the health professional with an understanding of the community context in which he or she is working. Questions may arise that will, in turn, lead to potential clarification through the structured needs and capacity assessment strategies. Social indicators also may support and supplement the results derived from the structured strategies.

Primary Data Collection

Primary needs and capacity assessment data are observations that the practitioner collects to make informed decisions regarding the next steps. Usually, these data complement and expand upon any secondary data collected from the work of others. Prior to the collection of primary data, human subjects' review should proceed through one's own organization or a partner organization (e.g., academic institution, medical center). Importantly, the protection of human subjects is the key consideration. This assurance should apply to individuals of all ages who will be offering information. The National Institutes of Health (NIH) has established very clear guidelines for those engaged in needs assessments (see the NIH Web site, *Human Participant Protections Education for Research Teams*: http://cme.nci.nih.gov). It usually will be necessary to have a proposal reviewed by an Institutional Review Board (IRB), which follows the NIH guidelines in analyzing the proposal. While the IRB process is important for the protection of all human subjects, it is even more imperative for those who are younger than 18 years of age or who have particular impairments. Researchers who are working with organizations that do not have their own IRB processes can check with local post-secondary education, medical, and/or human service institutions regarding the IRB processes they may have in place. This approach is particularly a reasonable one to follow when such agencies are involved in the assessment/planning process in a collaborative manner.

The strategies presented in the following chapters provide methods for the collection of primary data. Underlying all data collection procedures is the idea that observations must be collected in an accurate and consistent fashion. To accomplish this goal, the following considerations need to be addressed when planning the assessment approach.

Validity and Reliability

Validity refers to measuring what one purports to be measuring. It deals with the accuracy of the assessment process in detecting observations based on the principles and concepts underlying the measurement intent. Another measurement consideration closely aligned with validity is *reliability,* which refers to the consistency of the assessment process. Excellent extended discussions regarding validity and reliability in health education/health promotion contexts are provided by Baumgartner, Strong, and Hensley (2002), Green and Kreuter (1999), and Green and Lewis (1986).

Typically, validation procedures are used in developing measurement instruments for accurate data collection in research and evaluation efforts. Additionally, one can conduct a review of internal validity (i.e., observed program effects are based on an intervention) and external validity (i.e., ability to generalize the observed effects to similar populations). Research and evaluation procedures for assuring reliability relate primarily to the internal consistency (i.e., intercorrelations of all instrument items) or the stability (i.e., measurement association over time) of a measurement instrument. The resulting instruments then can be used in formative evaluation efforts (measurements before or during an intervention) and summative evaluation efforts (measurements regarding intervention impact). Because of the measurement's use with summative evaluation, "the stakes are higher for measurement error" (Green and Lewis, 1986, p. 121). For this reason, greater precision in validity and reliability determinations is required.

Needs assessments are used to detect and depict the perceived and actual needs of a given population so that realistic health education/health promotion objectives can be formulated. Capacity assessments typically are system-related resource review endeavors. Both types of assessments are more formative in nature. When instruments (e.g., surveys, wellness inventories, health risk appraisals) are to be used in needs and capacity assessments, validity and reliability concerns should be addressed. Chapter 3 discusses validity and reliability as they relate to survey development. For non-instrument formats (e.g., group assessments such as the nominal group and focus group processes), validity is the only factor of the two that can realistically be addressed.

Remember that needs and capacity assessment formats are used for the determination of needs and resources, not primarily for the research and evaluation of intervention impacts. For these purposes, we would recommend a validation procedure that incorporates the review of an advisory and/or expert group. Here individuals who are most familiar with the target population and some of its basic characteristics and issues can respond to the proposed process and make suggestions for improvement. This approach to validation then could be considered similar to the content validation process, in which experts are used in the development of research and evaluation instruments.

Sampling

Because it usually will be impossible to involve everyone from a given group in a needs and capacity assessment process, establishing a population sample is generally a more realistic approach. Samples are classified as *probability* samples, in which all individuals have an equal probability of being selected for the sample (e.g., simple random sample), or *nonprobability* samples, in which subject selection is based on key characteristics in a population (e.g., heterogeneous sample). An excellent in-depth discussion of these sample categories is provided by Green and Lewis (1986), including the justifications for using a given sampling approach. In addition, Creswell (2003) presents a very practical research design overview that differentiates qualitative, quantitative, and mixed methods (i.e., combining qualitative and quantitative approaches) for the collection and analysis of data. For many locally based needs and capacity assessment efforts that are not meant to have the results projected widely, the nonprobability sampling approach should be sufficient. In instances where it is imperative that the sample be truly representative of a larger population, probability sampling would be the approach of choice.

Needs and Capacity Analysis and Prioritization

Once data are collected through the secondary sources and/or through the structured strategies (to be detailed in forthcoming chapters), analyses of the meaning of the data must take place. It is strongly recommended that these procedures be established prior to the collection of the data, as part of the overall needs and capacity assessment plan. Because much of the information collected may be qualitative in nature, it is helpful to review in advance data analysis procedures for qualitative research methods. A succinct and practical overview is provided by Morse and Field (1995), who discuss the four cognitive processes of qualitative research: *comprehending* (clearer understanding of the circumstances being studied), *synthesizing* (aggregation of information), *theorizing* (finding the "best fit" explanation for the collected information), and *recontextualizing* (theory generalized into different settings). In each of the subsequent chapters, we address specific analytic procedures in the sections entitled "Using the Results."

Another important process in analyzing the collected information is prioritization. This analysis should be based on the needs and resources of the target group, as well as those of the population's service providers. The simplest method of prioritizing is to have the assessed needs and necessary resources ranked by target group members and representatives. In this process, individuals are asked to rank the top five (or some other predetermined number) needs and/or needed resources, out of all of those presented. In analyzing the group results, each need and/or resource has the potential of receiving a series of rankings, which can subsequently be averaged for a mean rank, or weighted. For example, in a 1–5 scale, a rank of 1 will have a weighting of 5; a rank of 2 will have a weighting of 4; and so forth. The weights are then added together for each need, with the highest-valued need being top ranked. We present an example of such assessments with multiple groups in the case study by Becker and Wabaunsee in Part V.

Due to the complexity of needs and capacities that can be assessed through various strategies, no one analytic process can serve all purposes. Thus, for more in-depth discussions regarding selected procedures, one may wish to review Doyle and Ward (2001, pp. 147–149), McKenzie and Smeltzer (1997, pp. 52–53), Dever (1991, pp. 45–73), McKillip (1987, pp. 105–119), and Witkin (1984, pp. 206–240).

A helpful model developed by Sork (1982) at the University of British Columbia is reviewed by Witkin (1984, pp. 230–232). This model offers a systematic process for determining priorities with a certain degree of built-in flexibility. The basic steps include the following:

1. *Select appropriate criteria.* Two general categories of importance and feasibility are suggested. Examples of importance are the number of people affected, the magnitude of the difference between present and future status, and the alignment with organizational goals. Examples of feasibility are efficacy levels of health education and promotion interventions (i.e., degree of benefit for those receiving the intervention), resource availability, and perceived ability to change.
2. *Assign a relative importance to each criterion.* Criteria are weighted equally or by degree on a scale of 1 to 10. The criterion of least weight (1) is identified first, and each subsequent criterion compared against it, so that the criterion weighted 10 is ten times the weight of 1.
3. *Apply each criterion to each need.* A separate list of priorities is established for each criterion used, with priority values expressed numerically or through descriptors such as high, medium, and low.
4. *Combine individual values to yield a total priority value for each need.* One approach here is to add weighted ranks and establish mean ranks for each identified need.
5. *Arrange needs from highest to lowest total priority value and indicate how priorities will be used.* Resource alignment with the identified needs can be established in this step.

From another vantage point, some decision makers may wish to review the assessed needs and resources in a highly qualitative fashion. Using this approach, special criteria can be established as questions against which the needs and resources will be reviewed through group discussion. Examples of such questions are offered in a manual published by the Ministry of Education in Victoria, British Columbia (Lund and McGechaen, 1981, pp. 16–17), and reviewed by Witkin (1984, p. 230):

- Does the target group recognize this need?
- How many people are affected?
- What would be the consequences if this need is not met?
- Can this need be met by an educational activity?
- Does this need coincide with your department or institution's program policies? If not, what are the reasons for the present policies? What procedures are available for influencing needed change?
- Can you rely on co-sponsorship or cooperation with another agency?
- Is this a critical need that should be met before other educational needs are addressed?
- Will resources (funds, staff) be adequate to meet those needs?

Using this approach, health professionals have the opportunity to discuss multiple responses to the questions, as well as the various rationales for those responses. While this approach typically takes more time, the complexity of the issues being addressed could well merit it.

Yet another prioritization approach has been advanced by Green and Kreuter (1999, p. 104) based on a series of questions during their phase of **epidemiological assessment:**

- Which problem has the greatest impact in terms of death, disease, days lost from work, rehabilitation costs, disability (temporary and permanent), family disorganization, and cost to communities and agencies for damage repair or loss and recovery?
- Are certain subpopulations—such as children, mothers, ethnic minorities, refugees, or indigenous populations—at special risk?
- Which problems are most susceptible to intervention?
- Which problem is not being addressed by other agencies in the community?
- Which problem, when appropriately addressed, has the greatest potential for an attractive yield in terms of improved health status, economic savings, or other benefits?
- Are any of the health problems highly ranked as a regional or national priority?

The results of needs and capacity assessments can guide the practitioners into the planning phases of program development. Key questions should serve as a guide, and those suggested by MacDonald et al. (2001) are particularly straightforward:

- What is the health problem and its consequences for the state or community?
- What is the size of the problem overall and in various segments of the population?
- What are the determinants of the health problem?
- Who are the target groups?
- What changes or trends are occurring? (p. 22)

In seeking the information needed to address these questions, MacDonald and colleagues recommend the use of secondary health status data at the national and state levels, particularly for specific groups. They encourage the assessment of capacity and infrastructure issues that can serve as indicators of issues needing to be addressed (e.g., disparities). Examples of capacity and infrastructure issues include the availability of researchers and research data and the availability of effective programs, community leadership, organizations, and networks.

Taken as a whole, these approaches assist the practitioner in keeping in mind the big picture of external forces and resources, as more delimited issues for a given target population (e.g., socioeconomic influences on youth tobacco use) are being assessed and reviewed for resolution.

Summary

The context of a practitioner's program planning experiences, observations, and secondary information sources provides a valuable framework for active involvement in health education and health promotion. This context also enables the professional to make decisions about more appropriate next steps for structured needs and capacity assessment strategies. Chapters 3 through 12 will detail these strategies by addressing selection considerations, along with preparation, implementation, and follow-up procedures.

Online Resources

Visit http://healtheducation.jbpub.com/gilmore for links to these Web sites.

American Journal of Health Promotion
Defines health promotion and the dimensions of health.

Public Health in America
Explains public health and the services and responsibilities of the profession, which include assessments, policy development, and assurance.

World Health Organization
The definition of health. Describes the strategic approach methodology, the first step of which is the strategic assessment.

The Urban Institute
Describes capacity and needs assessments of youth services in the District of Columbia.

HealthyPeople.gov
Healthy People 2000 publications broken down into documents and sections.

Western Rural Development Center
Outlines community assessment techniques. This site includes participant observation, social network analysis, the Delphi survey, the nominal group process, advisory groups, community forums, and application of these techniques.

Wisconsin Department of Public Instruction
Provides guidance through the Safe and Drug-Free Schools program, which includes the importance of needs assessments.

National Academies Press
Provides reference material regarding public health recommendations for the twenty-first century by the Institute of Medicine.

Community Tool Box
The Community Tool Box, sponsored by the University of Kansas, is designed to provide examples of assessment tools and guidance frameworks (e.g., logic model) to practitioners and community groups involved in planning, implementing, and evaluating health enhancement opportunities. A Tool Box search engine also is provided to assist in locating specific assessments within the Web site.

References

Bartholomew, L., Parcel, G., Kok, G., and Gottlieb, N. (2001). *Intervention Mapping*. Mountain View, CA: Mayfield Publishing.

Baumgartner, T., Strong, C., and Hensley, L. (2002). *Conducting and Reading Research in Health and Human Performance*. New York: McGraw-Hill.

Bensky, J., and Hietbrink, R. (1994). Getting Down to Business. *Worksite Health*, 1, 25–28.

Bond, L., Glover, S., Godfrey, C., Butler, H., and Patton, G. (2001). Building Capacity for System-Level Change in Schools: Lessons from the Gatehouse Project. *Health Education and Behavior*, 28, 368–383.

Bracht, N., and Gleason, J. (1990). Strategies and Structures for Citizen Partnerships. In Bracht, N. (Ed.), *Health Promotion at the Community Level* (pp. 109–124). Newbury Park, CA: Sage Publications.

Breslow, L. (1999). From Disease Prevention to Health Promotion. *JAMA*, 281, 1030–1033.

Butterfoss, F., Goodman, R., and Wandersman, A. (1993). Community Coalitions for Prevention and Health Promotion. *Health Education Research*, 8, 315–330.

Campbell, V., Crews, J., Moriarty, D., Zack, M., and Blackman, D. (1999). Surveillance for Sensory Impairment, Activity Limitation, and Health-Related Quality of Life Among Older Adults—United States, 1993–1997. *Morbidity and Mortality Weekly Report*, 48, 131–156.

Committee on Assuring the Health of the Public in the 21st Century, Board on Health Promotion and Disease Prevention. (2003). *The Future of the Public's Health in the 21st Century*. Washington, DC: National Academies Press.

Creswell, J. (2003). *Research Design: Qualitative, Quantitative, and Mixed Methods Approaches*. Thousand Oaks, CA: Sage Publications.

Cromley, E., and McLafferty, S. (2002). *GIS and Public Health*. New York: Guilford Press.

Dever, G. (1991). *Community Health Analysis: Global Awareness at the Local Level*. Gaithersburg, MD: Aspen Publishers.

Dewar, T. (1997). *A Guide to Evaluating Asset-Based Community Development: Lessons, Challenges, and Opportunities*. Chicago: ACTA Publications.

Doyle, E., and Ward, S. (2001). *The Process of Community Health Education and Promotion*. Mountain View, CA: Mayfield Publishing.

Florin, P., Mitchell, R., and Stevenson, J. (1993). Identifying Training and Technical Assistance Needs in Community Coalitions: A Developmental Approach. *Health Education Research*, 8, 417–432.

Gebbie, K., Rosenstock, L., and Hernandez, L. (Eds.) (2003). *Who Will Keep the Public Healthy? Educating Public Health Professionals for the 21st Century*. Washington, DC: National Academies Press.

Gilmore, G. D., and Hartigan, J. M. (1998). *Results of the April 1998 Rotary 3-H Health Planning Assessment in Dubna, Russia*. La Crosse, WI: Gundersen Lutheran Medical Center.

Green, L. (1999). Health Education's Contributions to Public Health in the Twentieth Century: A Glimpse Through Health Promotion's Rear-View Mirror. *Annual Review of Public Health*, 20, 67–88.

Green, L., and Kreuter, M. (1999). *Health Promotion Planning: An Educational and Ecological Approach*. Mountain View, CA: Mayfield Publishing.

Green, L., and Lewis, F. (1986). *Measurement and Evaluation in Health Education and Health Promotion*. Palo Alto, CA: Mayfield Publishing.

Green, L., and Raeburn, J. (1990). Contemporary Developments in Health Promotion. In Bracht, N. (Ed.), *Health Promotion at the Community Level* (pp. 29–44). Newbury Park, CA: Sage Publications.

Harvard Family Research Project. (2002). *Learning from Logic Models in Out-of-School Time*. Cambridge, MA: Author.

Hennessy, C., Moriarty, D., Zack, M., Scherr, P., and Brackbill, R. (1994). Measuring Health-Related Quality of Life for Public Health Surveillance. *Public Health Reports,* 109, 665–672.

Hunkeler, E., Davis, E., McNeil, B., Powell, J., and Polen, M. (1990). Richmond Quits Smoking: A Minority Community Fights for Health. In Bracht, N. (Ed.), *Health Promotion at the Community Level* (pp. 278–303). Newbury Park, CA: Sage Publications.

Joint Committee on Health Education and Promotion Terminology. (2001). Report of the 2000 Joint Committee on Health Education and Promotion Terminology. *American Journal of Health Education,* 32, 90–103.

Kretzmann, J., and McKnight, J. (1993). *Building Communities from the Inside Out.* Chicago: ACTA Publications.

Kretzmann, J., McKnight, J., and Puntenney, D. (1998). *A Guide to Creating a Neighborhood Information Exchange: Building Communities by Connecting Local Skills and Knowledge.* Chicago: ACTA Publications.

Kretzmann, J., McKnight, J., and Sheehan, G. (1997). *A Guide to Capacity Inventories: Mobilizing the Community Skills of Local Residents.* Chicago: ACTA Publications.

Lund, B., and McGechaen. (1981). *Continuing Education Programmer's Manual.* Victoria, British Columbia: Continuing Education Division, Ministry of Education.

MacDonald, G., Starr, G., Schooley, M., Yee, S., Klimowski, K., and Turner, K. (2001). *Introduction to Program Evaluation for Comprehensive Tobacco Control Programs.* Atlanta, GA: USDHHS, Centers for Disease Control and Prevention.

McKenzie, J., and Smeltzer, J. (1997). *Planning, Implementing, and Evaluating Health Promotion Programs: A Primer.* Boston: Allyn and Bacon.

McKillip, J. (1987). *Need Analysis: Tools for the Human Services and Education.* Beverly Hills, CA: Sage Publications.

Mokdad, A., Marks, J., Stroup, D., and Gerberding, J. (2004). Actual Causes of Death in the United States, 2000. *JAMA,* 291, 1238–1245.

Morse, J., and Field, P. (1995). *Qualitative Research Methods for Health Professionals.* Thousand Oaks, CA: Sage Publications.

Noack, H. (1987). Concepts of Health and Health Promotion. In Abeline, T., Brzezinski, Z., and Carstairs, V. (Eds.), *Measurement in Health Promotion and Protection.* Geneva: World Health Organization.

Parrish, R., and McDonnell, S. (2000). Sources of Health-Related Information. In Teutsch, S., & Churchill, R., (Eds.), *Principles and Practice of Public Health Surveillance.* New York: Oxford University Press.

Pellmar, T., Brandt, E., and Baird, M. (2002). Health and Behavior: The Interplay of Biological, Behavioral, and Social Influences: Summary of an Institute of Medicine Report. *American Journal of Health Promotion,* 16, 206–219.

Robertson, A., and Minkler, M. (1994). New Health Promotion Movement: A Critical Examination. *Health Education Quarterly,* 21, 295–312.

Shi, L. (1997). *Health Services Research Methods*. New York: Delmar Publishers.

Sork, T. (1982). *Determining Priorities*. Vancouver, British Columbia: University of British Columbia.

Teutsch, S., and Churchill, R. (2000). *Principles and Practice of Public Health Surveillance*. New York: Oxford University Press.

Timmreck, T. (2003). *Planning, Program Development, and Evaluation: A Handbook for Health Promotion, Aging, and Health Services*, 2nd ed. Boston: Jones and Bartlett Publishers.

U.S. Department of Health and Human Services (USDHHS). (2003). *A Public Health Action Plan to Prevent Heart Disease and Stroke*. Atlanta, GA: USDHHS, Centers for Disease Control and Prevention.

U.S. Department of Health and Human Services (USDHHS). (February 2001). *Healthy People in Healthy Communities: A Community Planning Guide Using Healthy People 2010*. Washington, DC: USDHHS, Office of Disease Prevention and Health Promotion.

U.S. Department of Health and Human Services (USDHSS). (January 2001). Health-Related Quality of Life among Persons with Epilepsy. *Morbidity and Mortality Weekly Report, 50*, 24–35.

U.S. Department of Health and Human Services (USDHHS). (November 2000). *Measuring Healthy Days: Population Assessment of Health-Related Quality of Life*. Atlanta, GA: USDHHS, Centers for Disease Control and Prevention.

U.S. Department of Health and Human Services (USDHHS). (May 2000). Health-Related Quality of Life among Adults with Arthritis—Behavioral Risk Factor Surveillance System, 11 States, 1996–1998. *Morbidity and Mortality Weekly Report, 49*, 366–369.

U.S. Department of Health and Human Services (USDHHS). (April 2000). Community Indicators of Health-Related Quality of Life—United States, 1993–1997. *Morbidity and Mortality Weekly Report, 49*, 281–285.

U.S. Department of Health and Human Services (USDHHS). (January 2000). *Healthy People 2010: Understanding and Improving Health*. Washington, DC: Author.

Wallerstein, N. (1992). Powerlessness, Empowerment, and Health: Implications for Health Promotion Programs. *American Journal of Health Promotion, 6*, 197–205.

Webb, K., Hawe, P., and Noort, M. (2001). Collaborative Intersectoral Approaches to Nutrition in a Community on the Urban Fringe. *Health Education and Behavior, 28*, 306–319.

Witkin, B. (1984). *Assessing Needs in Educational and Social Programs*. San Francisco: Jossey-Bass Publishers.

Working Group on Concepts and Principles of Health Promotion. (1987). Health Promotion: Concepts and Principles. In Abeline, T., Brzezinski, Z., & Carstairs, V. (Eds.), *Measurement in Health Promotion and Protection*. Geneva: World Health Organization.

World Health Organization. (1985). *Basic Documents*. Geneva.

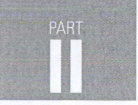

Assessments with Individuals

The three chapters in this section address the needs and capacity assessment strategies that can be used with individuals. The strategies incorporate the use of surveys and the process of interviewing. While many survey approaches involve just one contact with the participants, we also will describe the use of the Delphi process, which includes multiple contacts with the same participants on an individual basis. After reviewing each strategy, suggestions are offered for preparing and conducting the needs and capacity assessment processes, and then using the results in the planning process.

Single-Step Surveys

Introduction

Surveys are one of the oldest methods for gathering information. Face-to-face surveys date back to the ancient world. The Bible records a census of the Israelites, and the Roman Empire was conducting a census when Christ was born. The first "mail survey" may have been King Philip II of Spain's census of New World possessions, conducted by official courier in 1577 (Erdos, 1983, pp. 1–2). The invention of the telephone eventually led to the popularity of telephone surveys in the latter decades of the twentieth century.

Surveys have come a long way since these early examples. Today they are widely used, and we have all participated in them. At first, face-to-face surveys were preferred, as they could include a more representative cross section of the population (Fowler, 2002, p. 75).

Telephone surveys were initially considered unreliable. Because not all homes had phones, telephone surveys tended to include primarily educated and at least middle-income people.

Today's phone surveys can provide more reliable and valid information and may be the preferred method at this time (Fowler, 2002, p. 75). The telephone has become standard equipment in American households. Although unlisted numbers are increasing, "no call" lists are emerging, and more than half the phones in the world are now cellular, random-digit dialing and other similar techniques can enable surveyors to reach individuals who opt out of directory listings.

The rapid growth of the Internet in recent years has opened a new way of conducting surveys. A brief survey can be conducted using e-mail, or a longer survey can be posted on the World Wide Web for participants to complete. Internet surveys may become the preferred method of data collection in the years ahead, especially given that people are becoming more and more reluctant to participate in telephone surveys.

We define a *survey* as a structured process for collecting primarily quantitative data directly from individuals by asking questions. It can show the distribution of certain characteristics within a population, usually by surveying only a small portion of that population (Fowler, 2002, pp. 1–2).

Surveys have been widely used to assess educational needs. Mailing a questionnaire is probably the most frequently used strategy, and telephone surveys are also popular for this purpose. Face-to-face surveys have continuing importance for community health education, and Internet surveys are increasingly used as well. In this chapter we will discuss all four strategies.

You can learn to conduct good surveys, and you do not have to be an expert researcher to do so. You can follow the steps we outline in this chapter and obtain good results.

Reviewing and Selecting a Strategy

Mail Surveys

Advantages

Low cost. All surveys have similar basic costs, which include developing and producing the questionnaire, analyzing the data, and communicating the results. The cost of collecting data is the primary way costs differ among the various ways of conducting surveys. For mail surveys, the major data collection expense is postage. For many needs assessments, one person with a few basic research skills can conduct an entire mail survey from start to finish. Larger projects may require assistance from staff members with expertise in questionnaire design and data analysis, but one central office can handle the entire project.

Wide distribution. Mail surveys can reach anyone who receives mail from the postal service. You have relatively easy access to diverse groups of people.

Valid information. Mail surveys offer better chances of obtaining truthful answers than telephone or face-to-face surveys, especially when asking potentially threatening questions (Fowler, 2002, p. 64). People can respond in the privacy of their homes or workplaces. They do not have to muster the courage to talk to an interviewer.

Mail surveys provide opportunities to obtain thoughtful replies (Fowler, 2002, pp. 64, 73). Respondents can complete a survey when they have the time and perspective to give the best answers, rather than responding on the spot to an interviewer's questions. Mail surveys also eliminate the bias and influence that interviewers bring to telephone or face-to-face surveys.

Disadvantages

Lengthy process. Although mail surveys save money and personnel, time is lost while waiting for the return of the questionnaires. Data collection alone typically takes two months to complete (Fowler, 2002, p. 68), waiting for the returns from an initial mailing and subsequent follow-up efforts.

Limited number and type of questions. A lengthy questionnaire can discourage recipients from completing it. Simple and straightforward questions are most desirable. Complex questions are difficult to include, because you cannot follow up to clarify the meaning of responses.

No control over answers. You cannot control who answers your questionnaire. You may send it with explicit instructions for a teenager to complete, but you do not know whether she completed the survey or her father did. You cannot keep a respondent from consulting with another person before giving an answer. Nor can you encourage the respondent to answer all questions instead of skipping some.

Mailing list required. Complete mailing lists for a group you want to survey are not always readily available. If they are available, they may not be accurate. The more accurate lists may be expensive to obtain. Suddenly, what seemed to be an inexpensive survey becomes more costly.

Internet Surveys

Advantages
Lower cost. Internet surveys are even cheaper to conduct than mail surveys, because they eliminate the cost of postage. Assuming you have access to an Internet connection, distributing the survey is free. Some additional costs are possible for a Web survey, though, depending on your computer expertise. You may need assistance with posting the survey on the Web and retrieving the data received.

Shorter process. Communication between you and your participants is instantaneous. Compared to a mail survey, you save the time that the postal service needs to deliver your questionnaire to the respondents and then return the completed questionnaire to you. All follow-up contacts are delivered instantly as well. As with mail surveys, though, you still have to wait for respondents to take the time to complete the survey. People who actually complete an Internet survey may not wait as long as they would with a mail survey. Either they complete it relatively soon, or they forget about it (Dillman, 2000, pp. 366, 370).

Valid information. Internet surveys offer the same opportunity for obtaining truthful answers as mail surveys.

Higher response rate possible. These days, people may be more inclined to complete an Internet survey than a mail survey. It may be shorter and much quicker to fill out than a typical mail survey. Internet surveys are also more novel. People who resist completing one more mail survey may be willing to complete an Internet survey, simply because it is new and different.

Disadvantages
Limited distribution. Although the number of people in the United States with Internet access is growing rapidly, you simply cannot reach as many people as you would by regular mail.

Mailing list required. As with mail surveys, you need a list of e-mail addresses of people who fit the population you wish to sample. These days, we change our e-mail addresses more frequently than we change residences, so ensuring accuracy of the e-mail list is a major challenge. Using a mass e-mail distribution approach is not recommended. People respond very negatively to receiving mass-distributed e-mails and probably will not complete your survey. Instead, obtain a list of individuals who are likely to respond favorably to receiving an e-mail from you—for example, past program participants or people who have had some previous contact with your organization.

Potential sample bias. At the present time, people with Internet access tend to be better educated with higher incomes. An Internet survey may therefore exclude many less-educated lower-income people. Likewise, it may exclude many older people and the very young, as they typically have less access as well. Some people in these groups may use the Internet at public libraries or community agencies, but they would not have their own e-mail addresses so that you could invite them to participate in the survey.

Even more limited number and type of questions. An Internet survey needs to be shorter than a mail survey. A long computer document is more difficult for people to work with than a document they can handle physically. A well-designed Web survey can ask a number of questions, but you will need technical assistance to design it in a way that keeps respondents engaged. This technical assistance will add to the cost of your survey.

No control over answers. The same lack of control you have with mail surveys applies to Internet surveys as well.

Telephone Surveys

Advantages

More and different questions possible. Because talking is easier than writing, participants are typically willing to answer more questions for phone surveys than for mail or Internet surveys. For the general public, a survey lasting 10 to 20 minutes is reasonable. For relatively homogeneous groups of people, telephone surveys have lasted as long as 50 minutes or an hour with good results. Participants will tolerate open-ended questions much better over the phone than by mail. Complex questions are easier to ask, because follow-up questions are possible.

Better control over answers. Unlike with mail or Internet surveys, which are out of your hands once you drop them in the mail or hit the send button, you can make sure you are questioning the appropriate person. You can also discourage consultation with other people and encourage responses to all questions.

Shorter process. Preparation time for telephone surveys is slightly longer than for mail and Internet surveys, but data collection is quicker (Fowler,

2002, p. 68). You can call participants and have your information immediately. You do not have to wait two months or more for mail returns.

Good access to respondents. Although you can reach slightly fewer people by phone than by regular mail, a very high percentage of American households have access to a telephone. Random-digit dialing techniques can reach people with unlisted numbers (Fowler, 2002, pp. 23–25).

Immediate data entry. If resources permit, using computer-assisted telephone interviewing (CATI) makes data available in electronic format immediately following the interview. While more costly to set up, this approach reduces transcription errors and turnaround time.

Disadvantages

Response rate declining. People are becoming increasingly reluctant to participate in telephone surveys. Aided by caller identification features, they are hesitating to even answer their phones when they do not recognize the caller. When they do answer, they may quickly hang up if a pause occurs before the surveyor responds or decline to participate when they realize the purpose of the call. This behavior is partly a reaction to the increasing number of telemarketing calls at inconvenient times and partly a reflection of the increasing desire for privacy in our culture. Some people do not want to be bothered when they are at home.

Many states and the federal government have recently passed legislation creating "no-call" lists, which prohibits telemarketers from calling individuals who request not to be contacted. In many cases, this legislation applies to for-profit businesses, rather than nonprofit organizations. Even if your organization is not restrained from contacting people on a "no-call" list, these individuals may not respond favorably to your call.

More costly. Collecting data typically is more expensive than for mail or Internet surveys. If long-distance calls are necessary, they may cost more than postage to mail questionnaires. Conducting interviews is much more time-consuming than tracking mail or Internet surveys. For some telephone surveys, one person might conduct all of the interviews, but extra help is often needed. The additional interviewers may require payment for their training and interviewing time. For a large project involving several interviewers, supervisory help is needed as well.

Socially desirable responses. You have a better chance of receiving socially desirable responses to potentially threatening questions by phone than by mail or Internet (Fowler, 2002, p. 72). Candid answers are more easily written than stated to interviewers.

Face-to-Face Surveys

Advantages

Best opportunity for questioning. A face-to-face survey is the best way to administer a lengthy questionnaire (Fowler, 2002, p. 71). Open-ended and complex questions are best handled in face-to-face surveys, because follow-up questions are more easily asked.

Most control over answers. Compared to telephone surveys, you have even more assurance that the appropriate person is answering your questions and is not consulting with other people. Using both verbal and nonverbal expressions, you can also strongly encourage answering all questions.

Disadvantages

Most costly. Because interviewers must travel, often from house to house, to collect data, travel time and transportation expenses are significant. The interview itself typically takes longer to conduct in person than by phone. Although one person can carry out an entire mail or telephone survey, a face-to-face survey will require at least one other person to assist with interviews. Large projects require several interviewers as well as supervisory help. Training is more extensive, because interviewers must make judgments in the field without the benefit of consulting with a supervisor.

Socially desirable responses. Potentially threatening questions are the most difficult to ask in face-to-face surveys. Participants are most tempted to give a socially desirable answer when they have to face another person (Dillman, 2000, p. 226).

Difficulty in gaining access to participants. Historically, face-to-face surveys have offered good access to the public. As life has become busier and concerns about privacy and security have increased, however, face-to-face surveys have become more difficult to conduct. Many women have entered the workforce, leaving fewer people at home during the day. Families often have evening activities as well. Surveyors have increasing concerns about personal safety in some metropolitan neighborhoods, especially during evening hours, and more apartment buildings have installed security systems (Fowler, 2002, p. 66). Public places are also difficult for conducting surveys, because people are often in a hurry.

Criteria for Selection

As you consider the advantages and disadvantages of mail, Internet, telephone, and face-to-face surveys, we suggest you keep five criteria in mind: the type of information needed, from whom it is needed, the money available to conduct the survey, the time available, and the personnel who can assist you.

1. *Type of information.* If the information you need is potentially threatening to the participants, especially details about behavior patterns, a mail or Internet survey typically will yield more valid data. If you need to ask complex questions that require follow-up questions for clarification, a face-to-face survey offers the best opportunity. Open-ended questions are also best handled face-to-face. If you have

many questions to ask, a face-to-face survey is best, followed by a telephone survey.

2. *Audience.* If you plan to survey lower-income people, particularly low-literacy people or those not skilled in the use of English, a face-to-face survey usually is best (Fowler, 2002, p. 61). These individuals may be unable to complete a mail survey and may not feel comfortable talking to a stranger on the phone. For a professional audience, however, a telephone survey is more feasible. Professional people are comfortable using the phone and may resist completing one more mail survey. An Internet survey is an increasingly appropriate way to reach a professional audience. E-mail addresses for professionals at their place of employment are often relatively easy to obtain. Professional people make frequent use of their computer and the Internet and can complete the survey at times convenient for them.

3. *Money.* If money is tight, mail and brief Internet surveys are your best options. A simple telephone survey, however, can be inexpensive, as long as many long-distance calls are not required.

4. *Time.* If you need the survey done quickly, use the telephone or develop a brief e-mail survey. Note that if you use the phone, you will need time to recruit and train interviewers.

5. *Personnel.* A mail or brief e-mail survey requires the smallest number of personnel, while a face-to-face survey requires the largest number. A face-to-face survey also requires the most-qualified interviewers, because they are on their own when conducting the survey.

Finally, keep two other important considerations in mind, no matter which survey method you use to assess needs. First, remember that people respond based on how they feel at the time of the survey. They will not necessarily take action to meet their perceived needs at a later time. Second, remember that surveys have been widely used to assess needs. What once was novel is now potentially overused.

Preparing for the Assessment

Because the preparation phase is similar for mail, Internet, telephone, and face-to-face surveys, we will discuss the steps that apply generally to all four strategies. For some steps we will suggest considerations applicable to a particular survey method.

Decide What You Want to Know

Determine exactly what you need to learn from the individuals you plan to survey. Having a clear idea before you begin can direct development of your questions and save valuable time for both you and your participants.

Decide whether you need to ask people what they know, what their attitudes are about a certain subject, or how they would describe certain behaviors. If you plan to ask about behavior, consider whether describing this behavior will be threatening to the individual. With this in mind, plan for Institutional Review Board (IRB) review, to include informed consent considerations (Schiff, 2003).

Develop a Budget

Before you begin to develop a survey, you need to know how much money you can spend. You will already have an approximate budget in mind, which helped you select which survey method to use. Now put the budget in final form, including personnel costs for developing the questionnaire and collecting and analyzing the data, printing of the survey and final report, postage, long-distance telephone calls, travel expenses, and computer analysis. Having a detailed budget will help you decide, for example, how many people to employ, how many people to survey, and how much data analysis to do.

Prepare Your Questions

Before rushing ahead to develop your own questions, consider whether someone else has previously developed questions you could use. For a needs assessment, existing questions that fit your situation exactly may be difficult to find. With some modification, however, they might be suitable. Alternatively, they might suggest other questions you can develop yourself.

When developing questions, keep in mind which type of survey you plan to use, who you will survey, and how you will analyze the data you collect. Align your questions directly with the survey objectives. Remember that a mail survey should include primarily "closed" questions, which give the respondent a choice of answers to select. Examples include responding yes or no, indicating how frequently a certain situation applies, or rank ordering several possibilities.

"Open-ended" questions require participants to generate answers themselves. For a mail survey, limit the number of open-ended questions. The shorter the answer required, the better. An Internet survey offers more potential for open-ended questions, because using a computer to generate narrative responses is faster and easier than putting pen to paper. Telephone and face-to-face surveys can handle more plentiful and less focused open-ended questions.

The people you survey will also affect the type of questions you plan to develop. If you plan to survey a sample of the general public, remember that many will not be highly motivated to participate. Usually, they will respond better to closed questions than to open-ended ones. They may also refuse to answer threatening questions about their behavior.

If you plan to survey people who are highly motivated to participate, perhaps because they identify with your efforts or have a stake in the outcome, open-ended questions are more appropriate. These individuals will take more time to respond in a thoughtful manner.

How you plan to analyze your data should also influence the questions you develop. Open-ended questions may yield excellent information, but they take much more time and skill to analyze. If you are short on time, money, or skilled personnel, limit the number of open-ended questions.

Test and Modify Your Questions

After spending time and energy on developing questions, we all have a tendency to think we are finally ready to proceed with the survey. We may have some very good questions, but we need to submit them to careful scrutiny to make them even better. Taking time to revise your questions is the best way to decrease measurement error in responses, thereby increasing the reliability and validity of your survey.

We recommend at least the following steps. When developing your questions, seek to establish content validity by sharing them with colleagues who have experience with or expertise in the subject of the survey. Inform these people about the scope and purpose of your assessment, and have them use a consistent format in providing written feedback.

At this stage, other people can spot ambiguities or suggest alternate wording better than the developers can. Solicit the opinions of people who will analyze the data. Ask them to critique the questions and suggest ways to improve the wording. Ask them to tell you what they think the questions mean. Try not to worry about criticism of your questions. Think of them as first efforts, rather than polished masterpieces. Small changes in wording can influence how people respond. Revise your questions as many as ten times if necessary.

Develop a Draft of Your Survey

Keep your respondents in mind as you develop your questionnaire. Remember that they may have a low motivation to participate. Once they begin answering your questions, you want to ensure that they continue doing so. You do not want them to give up in the middle out of fatigue or frustration.

Start with questions that build interest in your survey and are relatively easy to answer. The first question is very important. It should apply to everyone, interest the respondent, and be easy to answer (Dillman, 2000, p. 92). Like a long-distance runner, the respondent needs to warm up and get into the flow of your survey. Use closed questions at this early stage, if at all possible.

Order your questions in a way that will seem logical to the respondent (Dillman, 2000, p. 88). Place difficult or potentially threatening questions near the middle. Open-ended questions also work best in the middle of the survey. You want the respondents to answer these questions after they are warmed up, but before they become tired.

Ask demographic or objectionable questions at the end (Dillman, 2000, p. 87). Questions about the respondent's age, income, and family status can scare off some respondents. Demographic questions are also answered quickly. When the finish line is in sight, having just a few quick questions left can help.

Continually ask yourself about the purpose of the assessment. Develop your questions while keeping this purpose ever-present in your mind. Many interesting questions are possible. The process of developing questions seems to encourage generating many questions. One question leads to another, just as in a good conversation. Once you have produced all these questions, however, ask yourself why you need the answer to each one. More importantly, ask yourself what you will do with the answer to each question.

If you have no specific use for the answer, or are not sure, omit the question. Do your participants a favor. They have to answer all your questions. The more questions you ask, the more fatigued they will become, and the more you risk having an incomplete survey or invalid information. Do yourself a favor, too. The more data you collect, the more you will have to summarize and analyze. You have only so much time and money to devote to this project, so use both wisely. Aim to have a few good questions.

Draft Coding and Data Analysis Procedures

Before pilot testing the survey, think through how you will analyze the data. Plan for statistical analysis, if appropriate. Consult with staff members who will handle the data analysis. They can suggest the best way to format the survey to make the data as easy to understand and categorize as possible.

Planning the data analysis procedures at this stage also ensures that it is done promptly. You could get so caught up in collecting data that the data could sit on the shelf too long before being used.

Pilot Test Your Survey

Be sure to allow enough time to conduct a pilot test. The time invested in this important preliminary activity should result in an effective format and increased response rate.

For a large research project, a rigorous regimen of pilot testing is strongly recommended to increase readability, reliability, and validity. Sudman and Bradburn (1983, p. 282) recommend several steps, including peer critique of a draft questionnaire, revision and testing with friends and colleagues, pilot testing with a small sample of respondents, written comments from interviewers and respondents, and pilot testing again.

If you cannot afford extensive pilot testing, at least find a group of people to practice taking your survey. Try to simulate the conditions to be used for the final version. Select a small sample of people, typically no more than 20, who are similar to those who will participate in the survey. Administer the practice survey, using the same directions you will use later. Include an extra page at the end for these pilot testers to comment about the questionnaire. Have them identify confusing questions and state the reasoning they used to answer them. Ask them to critique certain questions and suggest any improvements. Comments on the layout and format of the questionnaire are also useful.

This feedback about the questions themselves is important for large or small pilot-testing efforts. Determining what the questions mean to the respondents and ensuring that the questions elicit the responses you intend are important ways to increase validity. For more information about these "cognitive debriefing" approaches, see Tanur (1992).

Once you have received the completed pilot surveys, analyze the data just as you would with the final version. Determine as best you can whether the questions are providing the information you need and whether the coding and data analysis procedures are clear and effective.

Design the Final Survey

Consider three groups of people when designing the final questionnaire: the respondents, the interviewers (if used), and the data analysts.

For a *mail survey*, give the respondents primary consideration. Remember that length is important, especially for the general public. Generally, the shorter the survey and the simpler the questions, the better the responses. For the general public, try to limit your questionnaire to approximately four pages. For relatively homogeneous groups who identify with your project, however, longer surveys are feasible. Use only a few open-ended questions, if any.

The most important consideration is always that your survey be easy to read. Use a relatively large and legible typeface. Do not try to shorten the survey by reducing the type size. What you gain by having fewer pages, you will lose by having difficult-to-read type. A slightly longer survey, if you really need to ask all those questions, is better than a survey with type that is too small. Also, make sure you include good directions. If respondents must skip certain questions based on how other questions are answered, make sure these directions are clearly identified.

Design your mail survey to look as professional as possible, without being slick. Everything you do to design the questionnaire should be geared toward obtaining the best response for the money available. Use different fonts, variable type size, boldface, shading, and other word processing and desktop publishing enhancements to create an attractive, easily followed, low-cost survey. If the budget allows, designing an attractive booklet with a cover page, preferably printed on legal size paper folded to become a 8.5×7 inch booklet, can increase responses (Dillman, 2000, pp. 81–83, 102–108).

An *e-mail survey* typically consists of a brief set of questions included in the e-mail message. Participants insert their responses into the message and return it to the sender. Some people are more comfortable working with paper and pen, so offer them the option of printing a copy, marking their responses on the hard copy, and returning it via regular mail.

Simplicity is key for an e-mail survey. Limit the number of questions to as few as three to five (Dillman, 2000, p. 372). Because many people tend to delete e-mail messages after reading just a few lines, make sure the first question is especially interesting to the respondents. Use the first question to pique their interest and encourage completion of the survey. Use bracket symbols ([ ]) to indicate where they should place their responses. Brackets are not frequently used in narrative writing and will tend to stand out for the respondent (Dillman, 2000, pp. 370–371).

Because respondents will have different computers and e-mail programs, an e-mail questionnaire can appear differently on their computer screens than it does on yours. A question that fits on one line on your screen may extend to two lines on a respondent's screen, making the questionnaire less attractive and more confusing to complete. Keep lines as short as possible to avoid this "wraparound" effect (Dillman, 2000, p. 369–370).

A *Web survey* offers several opportunities not available with an e-mail survey. You can dress up the questionnaire with color, attractive graphics, or pictures. These features enable you to include questions that require respondents to view a picture or diagram and answer questions about it. A Web survey also offers a better opportunity to use open-ended questions than a mail or e-mail survey. People are more inclined to generate narrative responses to open-ended questions when using their computer than when putting pen to paper. A Web survey can also be longer than an e-mail survey, as there are various ways to sustain interest.

Keep the survey on continuous scrolling, rather than using a method that requires exiting from one page to another. Continuous scrolling allows respondents to mark their progress in completing the survey (Dillman, 2000, pp. 395–396). Allow respondents to skip questions they do not wish to answer, rather than forcing them to answer each question before proceeding to the next. If respondents are forced to answer all questions, they may stop working on the survey if they are asked a question they do not wish to answer. Forcing respondents to answer all questions can also introduce bias, because mail, e-mail, telephone, and face-to-face surveys all allow respondents to skip questions (Dillman, 2000, p. 394).

Although a Web survey offers many attractive possibilities, exercising restraint is key. Many respondents may not have computers as powerful or Internet connections as fast as you do, especially if they are completing their surveys at home. If you make extensive use of color, graphics, and pictures, respondents' computers may be unable to load them. Or their computers may take so long for the screen to be complete, that they become frustrated and stop working on the survey. It is better to design a Web survey that will load quickly and completely on less powerful computers and slower Internet connections (Dillman, 2000, pp. 385–389).

The more elaborate the Web survey, the more likely you will need to pay for assistance in developing it. Thus the size of your budget will influence how fancy you make it as well.

For *telephone* and *face-to-face surveys,* give the interviewers primary consideration. A good design can help alleviate some of the pressure that is a normal part of conducting a survey. The length of the questionnaire is no longer as important. Instead, make sure you include clear directions and enough space to record answers. Design the booklet to be easy to use during the survey. Use extra white space to set the questions apart from one another.

As much as possible, design the survey to enhance good data analysis. Place the answers in a consistent location for easy reading. If the survey will be scored by a computer, include the appropriate field numbers. If the budget allows, consider using a software program that enables interviewers to enter data directly into a computer while conducting the survey.

Conducting the Assessment

Although the preparation phase is similar for mail, Internet, telephone, and face-to-face surveys, the conducting phase varies significantly. We will discuss the appropriate steps for each type.

Mail Survey

Select a Sample of Respondents

Unless you have a very small group of people to survey, you will have to sample from a larger population. A *probability sample* (defined in Chapter 2) is usually the best option in this case. A mail survey enables you to obtain information about educational needs from a comparatively large and potentially diverse group of people. Selecting a probability sample ensures that this information is representative of the population you want to serve.

In its simplest form, you can select a probability sample by drawing a *random sample* of names out of a hat. Alternatively, you can use a table of random numbers from a statistics text or computer program to select the required number of names from a mailing list (Salant and Dillman, 1994, pp. 61–63).

These pure forms of random selection, however, are not typically used in practice. Instead, a systematic sample, which in most cases is comparable to a random sample, is created by selecting names at regular intervals from a mailing list (Dillman, 2000, p. 210).

To obtain a *systematic sample,* first decide how many respondents you want to survey, and make sure your budget can handle this number. Then divide the number of names on the list by the size of the sample needed to determine the size of the interval between names to be selected. Pick a number at random between one and the size of the interval, inclusive. Draw this number from a hat or select it from a table of random numbers; it is the number of the first name selected from your mailing list. Skip as many names as the size of the interval and select that name. Proceed through the entire list to complete your sample, selecting names at each interval.

For example, if you want to select 50 participants from a mailing list of 500 people, the interval size is ten. Randomly select a number between one and ten, inclusive. If that number is seven, choose the seventh person on the list. Then choose the seventeenth person, the twenty-seventh person, and so on, through the entire list.

When conducting a survey, you may want to make sure that certain groups of people are adequately represented in the sample. For a survey of the health education needs of a particular community, for example, you will want to understand the needs of all age groups. If you rely exclusively on a telephone directory, voter registration records, or a list of motor vehicle licenses, your sample will include primarily working adults. To ensure representation from young people and older adults, seek other sources of information, such as school registration records and lists of individuals currently served by programs for seniors.

Once you have obtained appropriate lists that represent these different age groups, select a *stratified sample*. Divide the young people, working adults, and older people into three discrete groups, called strata, using the different mailing lists. Make sure that no one appears on more than one list. Then proceed to select systematic samples from each of these lists using the procedure described above. For each age group, try to make the sample size proportional to the population of that age group in the community.

Cluster sampling is another way to select representative groups using naturally occurring groups or clusters, such as schools, clinics, worksites, or census tracks. All, or a random selection of some, of the individuals in a cluster can be used depending on the intent of the assessment. In most instances, even though individuals are in close proximity in a cluster, there is sufficient variability or heterogeneity. Cluster sampling is particularly helpful when a list of group members is not available, when the population is spread over a large area, or when it is not convenient to remove selected individuals from their group to conduct the assessment. Keep in mind that conclusions and inferences drawn from the data need to include reference to the particular cluster sampled (Baumgartner, Strong, and Hensley, 2002).

Mail the Questionnaires

Include a brief cover letter that explains who is conducting the survey, why it is important, and what benefits will result from it. Explain how the respondents were selected, and note that their responses will be kept confidential. Code the questionnaires with a number in an inconspicuous place. That way you can tell who has and who has not responded. Assure the respondents that this number is just for coding purposes.

Indicate a date by which the respondents should return the questionnaire, typically two weeks. Busy people may not complete the survey right away, but you do not want it sitting around for so long they forget about it. Include a stamped, self-addressed or business-reply envelope for return of the survey.

You may also want to consider sending a letter to your sample a few days to a week in advance of mailing the survey. This letter alerts the sample members to the coming survey and seeks their cooperation in completing it.

If the project budget and organization policy allow, consider a small financial incentive to encourage participation in the survey. To counter growing resistance to surveys, especially from younger adults, including one or two dollars in the original mailing can increase response rate (Dillman, 2000, p. 168). If you are especially concerned about a low response rate, consider offering a small gift certificate for a major bookstore or franchise restaurant. While conducting a national survey, one of the authors (GDG) had a good response to entering respondents in a drawing for savings bonds and donated professional memberships and books.

Follow Up the Initial Mailing

Three additional contacts with potential respondents are recommended to increase the response rate (Dillman, 2000, pp. 156–188). Send a reminder postcard one week after mailing the survey. Two weeks later, mail a letter and another copy of the questionnaire to those people who have not responded. Wait another four weeks to contact individuals who still have not responded, perhaps using the telephone. If resources permit, offer to conduct the survey by phone for these nonrespondents. For all follow-ups, include investigator contact information for respondents to raise questions if desired.

At this point, your response rate may not be as high as you would like it to be. It is tempting to continue contacting people in an effort to increase the response. Always, however, maintain a balance between trying to increase the response rate as much as possible and bothering people to the point that they won't complete your survey anyway (Dillman, 2000, pp. 29, 187).

Internet Survey

In many ways, conducting an Internet survey is similar to conducting a mail survey. You need to develop an instrument, pretest it, obtain a mailing list, distribute the survey, and have follow-up contact. In other ways, though, an Internet survey differs from a mail survey.

Decide Who to Survey

Although the number of people in the United States with Internet access is growing rapidly, it remains much smaller than the number who have a telephone or receive mail from the postal service.

Because Internet access is more limited, selecting a sample that is representative of a particular population can pose a challenge. If you need to survey the general public, justifying an Internet survey as being representative of the population is difficult. If you plan to survey a professional population, however, you have a better chance of selecting a representative sample. Most professional groups have widespread Internet access, and e-mail addresses are relatively easy to obtain.

Because distributing an e-mail or Web survey is so easy and essentially free once you have an e-mail list, you may want to survey an entire population for some surveys instead of sampling.

Distribute the Survey

For an e-mail survey, sending a note before the survey is distributed is important. People can easily overlook or quickly delete an e-mail message. Sending a note two days in advance will alert the respondents to anticipate the survey and deter them from deleting it too quickly (Dillman, 2000, p. 368).

For a Web survey, you can distribute the survey with an e-mail message, embedding the Web address in the e-mail. Respondents can click on the Web address to get transferred to the survey. Alternatively, you can telephone or send a letter, directing respondents to the Web address to complete the survey. This latter approach is useful when you do not have access to an e-mail list.

Follow Up the Initial Distribution

Continue to have the same number of contacts with the e-mail/Web sample as with a mail survey, but shorten the interval of time between contacts. The first follow-up can include another copy of the questionnaire, because it is easy and inexpensive to distribute. All subsequent follow-ups can include a copy of the questionnaire as well (Dillman, 2000, pp. 367–368).

Telephone Survey

Select a Sample of Respondents

If you plan to survey employees or members of an organization, obtain the staff directory or membership list. Then draw a systematic sample from this population.

If you plan to survey the general public, the community telephone directory is the most obvious source of phone numbers. This directory, however, will not include unlisted numbers. Computer-assisted random-digit dialing is the best way to gain access to unlisted numbers, but a simple and effective method is to add a digit (Frey, 1989, pp. 90–104). Draw a systematic sample of telephone numbers, and then add one digit to every number. That way you are not limited to just phone numbers in the directory.

Gaining cooperation in completing the survey is a challenge when using random-digit dialing. There is often a delay after the respondent answers the phone until the interviewer begins to speak. This delay alerts the respondent that some kind of solicitation is about to occur, which typically results in a negative reaction.

Select and Train the Interviewers

Consider age and experience when recruiting interviewers. Older interviewers and interviewers with some experience may obtain better response rates than younger interviewers.

Explain the purpose of the survey, who is conducting it, why it is important, and what benefits will result from it. Give the interviewers written instructions on how to conduct the surveys. Specify how many attempts to make to reach a participant before proceeding to someone else, how to introduce the survey, how to handle ambiguous answers, and how to record the data.

Have the interviewers practice conducting telephone interviews and critique one another. If possible, have them contact people similar to the survey participants or have them practice on one another.

Collect and Record the Data

The interviewers simply proceed through the survey, following the directions on the questionnaire and the instructions they received during training. If possible, have all interviewers place calls from a central location during the same period of time. That way one supervisor can handle any problems that arise.

As noted earlier, using computer-assisted telephone interviewing (CATI) makes data available in electronic format immediately following the interview.

Weekday evenings from January through March have been shown to be the best times to conduct telephone interviews (Dillman, 2000, p. 176). People tend to spend more time at home in winter.

Face-to-Face Survey

Decide Who and Where to Survey

Various possibilities exist for conducting a face-to-face survey. You can select a systematic sample of participants from a membership list and arrange to survey them in person. You can also interview, for example, the oldest female member of every fifth household in a neighborhood, or randomly select people at a shopping mall or on a street corner.

A *cluster sample* is another way to obtain a probability sample for a face-to-face survey. First, divide the total population into natural groupings or clusters. To understand the health education needs of an entire community, for example, we might divide the community into neighborhoods, city blocks, or even types of nonprofit community organizations. Then randomly or systematically sample a certain number of respondents from within each cluster (Green and Lewis, 1986, p. 230).

Select and Train Interviewers

The selection of interviewers is more critical for a face-to-face survey than for a telephone survey. Interviewers need to enjoy and feel comfortable in a face-to-face situation. Because they will conduct these surveys with little or no supervision, they need to exercise good judgment. Once the interviewers are selected, training is similar to phone survey training.

Collect and Record the Data

Give the interviewers explicit instructions on who and where to survey. The data collection itself is similar to the telephone survey.

Using the Results

After a sustained preparation and data collection effort, you may prefer to set the data aside while you catch up with other projects. The momentum you have established to this point, however, is important to maintain. If you set the data aside now, you may have difficulty returning to the project later. Planning your data analysis earlier will help you keep going now, working through any slump that might occur.

Most of the data you collect from a survey will be quantitative data. You need some way to summarize these numbers for your planning committee or other interested groups. Sophisticated statistical tests typically are not necessary for a needs assessment. As discussed in Chapter 1, a needs assessment is not the same as rigorous academic research. Although some of the same research skills are used, the data are used differently.

Simple descriptive statistics are usually sufficient for a needs assessment. Do the following calculations.

1. *Tabulate frequency distributions.* Count the number of times each response occurs for each item. For a small survey, count these responses manually, or use a simple software spreadsheet program to summarize frequencies. For a large survey, enter response data into a computer to obtain frequency distributions.

2. *Determine the range of responses.* Note the lowest response and the highest response for each item.

3. *Calculate the most appropriate measure of central tendency.* The *mean*—the arithmetic average of all responses to the item—is used most often. It is appropriate when you have a relatively narrow range of responses with a relatively even distribution. To calculate the mean, add the scores and divide by the number of responses.

   Sometimes the median or the mode is a more helpful statistic. The *median* is most simply understood as the middle score in the distribution. It is a more appropriate measure of central tendency when a few scores are skewed much higher or much lower than the rest of the scores. To determine the median, arrange all responses in ascending order from low to high. Count the scores, beginning with the lowest score, until you reach the middle score. That is the median. If you have an even number of scores, determine the point halfway between the two middle scores (i.e., the average of these two scores).

The *mode* is the response that occurs most frequently. It is an appropriate measure of central tendency when one particular response to an item is clearly more frequent than any other.

Statistically, calculating the mean is appropriate when analyzing interval or ratio data (e.g., age levels). Determining the median is appropriate when analyzing ordinal data (e.g., strongly agree, agree, disagree, strongly disagree). The mode is appropriate for nominal data (e.g., yes or no).

Desktop computers have simple spreadsheet programs that can analyze data and compute these statistics for even small surveys.

Although most survey data are quantitative, some data may be qualitative. That is, you will have verbal responses to analyze instead of numbers. If you have surveyed only a few people, you can handle open-ended questions by simply listing verbatim the responses received. Typically, the open-ended questions from a survey will yield responses that are relatively short and to the point. Some respondents may add comments in the margins that you may want to summarize as well.

Another way to handle verbal responses, especially when you have a large number of participants, is to combine similar responses into more of a summary statement. Indicate how many people offered each type of response. Be careful not to collapse similar statements too much, such that you lose some of the meaning. The more you summarize, the more you introduce your own interpretation into the responses. You want to present the responses as faithfully as possible in the way they were received. Later, you can add your own interpretation.

If you have a variety of responses to a particular question, you may need to do more collapsing and interpreting. First, read quickly through all responses to the item to get a sense of the range of responses. Think of possible categories as you read, and jot them down. Next, develop an initial list of categories. Reread the responses, and count the responses that fit into each category. As you make this first attempt at categorizing responses, you may think of additional categories that fit the data better. Add these categories to your list, rather than forcing a response into a category that seems to distort the meaning. After completing this second reading of the data, consider combining similar categories or rearranging them in some way. Finally, some miscellaneous responses may not fit any category, so report them separately. After this qualitative analysis, you may want to report the results in some quantitative form. Use frequency tabulations, range, and measures of central tendency as appropriate.

The final step in this phase is to share the results with your planning committee or other interested groups. Remember that we cautioned earlier against collecting extraneous data. If you do collect too much data, you will spend too much time analyzing it. You might also give your planning committee too much information and confuse, rather than help, the planning process. Consider using graphics and PowerPoint presentations, which are readily available on desktop computer software programs (Dillman, 2000, pp. 95, 106).

Reviewing an Example

In addressing system-level change in schools in Victoria, Australia, through capacity building, Bond, Glover, Godfrey, Butler, and Patton (2001) described their multiple assessment efforts in the Gatehouse Project. In this school-based mental health promotion program, "the intervention is based on an understanding of individual and social risk processes for adolescent depression and emotional well-being" (p. 370). The authors focused on the school's social environment (e.g., bullying, conflict, isolation, alienation), as well as individual cognitive and social skills. To gather the necessary information, Bond et al. (2001) used a battery of process evaluation assessments, including field notes, key informant interviews, school background audits, and the Gatehouse Project Adolescent Health Questionnaire for student input. This particular survey was quite comprehensive in terms of assessing students' perceptions of social connectedness (e.g., levels of social interaction, school connectedness, issues of victimization), levels of anxiety and depression symptoms, degree of deliberate self-harm, and usage levels of tobacco, alcohol, and illicit drugs. Based on the assessments, realistic capacity-building interventions were developed from a whole-school approach.

Online Resources

Visit http://healtheducation.jbpub.com/gilmore for links to these Web sites.

American College Health Association
Describes the National College Health Assessment, including generalizability, reliability, and validity discussions.

National Network for Child Care
An example of a needs assessment for a school-aged childcare program.
An example of a nutrition assessment.

Western Rural Development Center
Outlines community assessment techniques. This site includes participant observation, social network analysis, the Delphi survey, the nominal group process, advisory groups, community forums, and application of these techniques.

Centers for Disease Control and Prevention
Description of the CDC's National Maternal and Infant Health Survey.

Wisconsin Department of Health and Family Services
Provides access to information on the Behavioral Risk Factor Survey and the Family Health Survey.

National Family Health Survey
Provides state and national information for India on fertility, infant and child mortality, the practice of family planning, maternal and child health, reproductive health, nutrition, anemia, and utilization and quality of health and family planning services.

Wisconsin's Information Network for Successful Schools (WINSS)
Examples of successful schools surveys from the Wisconsin WINSS program.

References

Baumgartner, T., Strong, C., and Hensley, L. (2002). *Conducting and Reading Research in Health and Human Performance,* 3rd ed. Boston: McGraw-Hill.

Bond, L., Glover, S., Godfrey, C., Butler, H., and Patton, G. (2001). Building Capacity for System-Level Change in School: Lessons from the Gatehouse Project. *Health Education and Behavior,* 28, 368–383.

Dillman, D. A. (2000). *Mail and Internet Surveys: The Tailored Design Method,* 2nd ed. New York: John Wiley & Sons.

Erdos, P. L. (1983). *Professional Mail Surveys.* Malabar, FL: Robert E. Krieger Publishing.

Fowler, F. J. (2002). *Survey Research Methods,* 3rd ed. Thousand Oaks, CA: Sage Publications.

Frey, J. H. (1989). *Survey Research by Telephone,* 2nd ed. Newbury Park, CA: Sage Publications.

Green, L. W., and Lewis, F. M. (1986). *Measurement and Evaluation in Health Education and Health Promotion.* Palo Alto, CA: Mayfield Publishing.

Salant, P., and Dillman, D. A. (1994). *How to Conduct Your Own Survey.* New York: John Wiley & Sons.

Schiff, L. (2003). *Informed Consent: Information, Production, and Ideology.* Lanham, MD: Scarecrow Press, Inc.

Sudman, S., and Bradburn, N. M. (1983). *Asking Questions: A Practical Guide to Questionnaire Design.* San Francisco: Jossey-Bass Publishers.

Tanur, J. M. (Ed.). (1992). *Questions about Questions: Inquiries into the Cognitive Bases of Surveys.* New York: Russell Sage Foundation.

Multi-Step Surveys: Delphi

Introduction

The Delphi Technique had its beginnings in the 1950s in a study done by the Rand Corporation for the United States Air Force, in which it was reasoned that one gets closer to the truth when there is the combined judgment of a large number of people. Its name derives from the Oracles at Delphi in ancient Greece, who would predict the future (Moore, 1987). In addition to forecasting, this approach can be used for the following purposes, as detailed by Moore (1987, p. 50): to identify goals and objectives, to examine possible alternatives, to establish priorities, to reveal group values, to gather information, and to educate a respondent group.

The Delphi Technique is a group process that generates a consensus through a series of questionnaires. Usually, the respondents are unable to meet in one place due to geographical or time limitations. The process typically involves three groups: decision makers, staff, and respondents (Delbecq, Van de Ven, and Gustafson, 1986). In some organizations, the decision makers and staff are the same group. The size of the respondent group varies, with 10 to 15 participants recommended for each representative group. A questionnaire consisting of one or two broad questions is sent out to the respondents. Their responses are analyzed, and from these a second questionnaire is developed. The respondents are then asked to answer more specific questions for further clarification. Their responses are again analyzed, and a third questionnaire is sent out asking for additional information. The process may end here or continue until a consensus is reached. Usually, the three to five rounds are necessary. The Delphi process aligns with the Social Diagnosis phase of the PRECEDE/PROCEED model (Green and Kreuter, 1999).

Reviewing the Strategy

Advantages

Pooled responses. The Delphi process draws from subjective responses and is appropriate in situations where objective information is not available from other sources.

Spans distance and time. People who are separated by geography or busy schedules can be involved. This ability to span distances and longer time frames is especially useful when trying to obtain expert opinion.

High motivation and commitment. Individuals who agree to participate in a Delphi study are usually highly motivated and committed, contributing a substantial amount of information.

Reduced influence by others. There is no face-to-face contact, which reduces conformity, domination, and/or conflict. Of note, participants can remain anonymous (Butler and Howell, 1996).

Enhanced response quality and quantity. The written-response format encourages an increase in both the quality and the quantity of ideas.

Equal representation. Participants' ideas are given equal representation through the synthesis.

Consistent participant contact. The feedback process enables the participants to respond throughout the study and have a sense of closure when the study is completed. This quality of the process is enhanced with the advent of computer-based Delphi processes. This approach presents the opportunity for continuous feedback, rather than being locked into a response round structure (Turoff and Hiltz, 1996).

Disadvantages

High cost and time commitment. A large amount of administrative time and high costs are involved. There is also a considerable time commitment on the part of the participants. Responding to the questionnaires may take ten hours or longer.

Reduced clarification opportunities. There are fewer opportunities to clarify the meanings of specific responses, which become open to the interpretation of the staff. Because the participants do not meet directly, there is no opportunity for clarification of comments or further discussion on areas of disagreement. Points of disagreement are synthesized rather than addressed or resolved (Gilmore, 1977).

Reduced immediate reinforcement. In comparison with needs assessment strategies that encourage direct participant interactivity, there are fewer immediate rewards for the respondents. Thus, they must be more inherently motivated to participate.

Preparing for the Assessment

At least 30 to 45 days should be allowed to prepare for the Delphi Technique. During this time the following tasks should be accomplished.

1. *Develop a workgroup.* The workgroup consists of staff and administrative people, and usually has five to nine members. They will develop and revise the questions, synthesize the responses, and determine the usefulness of the questionnaires.

2. *Assign a project manager.* This person should be experienced in the Delphi Technique and knowledgeable about the problem being explored. He or she will guide the workgroup.

3. *Enlist sufficient support staff.* You will need assistance in typing, mailing the questionnaires, and organizing the responses in a way that will facilitate the synthesis.

4. *Establish a timeline.* A timeline will be very helpful in keeping the project on schedule.

5. *Identify potential participants.* The workgroup or other people who are knowledgeable about the particular need area can generate a list or lists of people who can be contacted to obtain their participation in the Delphi exercise. These potential participants should be interested in your topic, knowledgeable about the topic, and motivated to complete the series of questionnaires. Depending on the scope of your needs assessment, the list for each representative group can range from 25 to 100 people or more.

6. *Clarify your goals and objectives.* If the decision makers of your organization are not directly involved in the Delphi process, it is important to clearly understand what they want to accomplish. Clarification of goals and objectives will help structure the questions and organize the results of each questionnaire.

Conducting the Assessment

Once the preliminary steps are completed, you are ready to begin the Delphi process. Conducting the Delphi process requires the following steps.

1. *Develop the first questionnaire and pretest it.* This step is crucial. The question(s) must be understandable to the respondents and generate the kind of information you are seeking. Have several members of the staff or representative groups review the question(s) for any needed clarity. The first questionnaire is generally broad in nature and simple in form, consisting of one or two open-ended questions, a request for

a list with examples, or some other format that will generate information that is relevant and manageable for further questionnaires.

2. *Choose the participants.* From the participant list or lists, individuals can be contacted and asked to nominate other respondents. Alternatively, the individuals can be randomly selected from the list(s). A total of 10 to 15 people should be selected for each representative group. More people may be selected if you are working with only one homogeneous group, although this number should not exceed 30 (Delbecq, Van de Ven, and Gustafson, 1986). Once the potential respondents have been identified, they should be contacted in person or by phone. Prior to asking for their involvement, they should be informed about the type of needs assessment, the purpose of the process, the composition of the respondent group(s), the time investment and commitment required on the part of each respondent, and the ways that the results will be shared. Depending on the complexity of the process, it may be necessary to convey detailed information in writing prior to asking for a commitment to be involved.

3. *Send out the questionnaire with a cover letter to the respondents.* This step should be done as soon as possible after the respondents have been contacted. Both the questionnaire and the cover letter should be well constructed and well designed. Along with expressing appreciation for participating in the study, the cover letter should briefly outline the points that were presented in the initial contact with the participant. A response date of two weeks should be emphasized, and a stamped, self-addressed envelope should be enclosed for ease in responding.

   To encourage a timely response, you may want to send a letter or postcard in the second week, reminding the participants of the response date. A phone call also may be necessary for the late respondents.

4. *Synthesize and analyze the responses to the first questionnaire.* As the questionnaires are returned, the responses can be recorded on a master list for ease in analysis. Once all questionnaires have been returned, call a meeting of the workgroup. Provide the members with a copy of the master list, which they can use to sort the items into similar categories. Each item can be placed on an index card and placed into a pile of similar items. Then, each pile can be labeled and the labeled categories listed and discussed until the group members reach a consensus regarding a final list. The items in the final list should next be summarized into clear and concise statements, which will make up the second questionnaire. Instead of using index cards, it would be very convenient to use a word processor for this, and subsequent, steps in the process.

5. *Develop and send out the second questionnaire.* The purpose of the second questionnaire is to get further clarification concerning the information gathered from the first questionnaire. It should provide an accurate summary of the results of the first questionnaire. Participants are asked to review, comment, clarify, and vote on each specific item listed in the summary from the first questionnaire. The process of developing the second questionnaire should follow the same steps as the first questionnaire. The format employed will depend on the kind of information obtained from the first questionnaire and the kind of additional information needed. Try to keep the new questionnaire short enough so that it can be completed in less than 30 minutes.

6. *Synthesize and analyze the responses to the second questionnaire.* The synthesis of the second questionnaire consists largely of a tally of the votes for each item. A tally sheet can be used that includes the list of items, the number of individuals voting for each item, the values of the individual votes, and the total vote. Comments should be summarized and then grouped with each item as in the first questionnaire.

7. *If necessary, develop and send out a third questionnaire.* Often, when a ranking of importance of each item is desired, a third questionnaire can be developed and sent out. It provides for achieving additional consensus as well as closure for the participants. The questionnaire should be designed to enable the participants to review a summary of previous comments and the results of the first vote for each item under consideration. A final ranking or vote plus any additional comments can be requested. The procedure for developing and sending out the questionnaire is the same as for the questionnaires discussed previously.

8. *Synthesize and analyze the responses to the third questionnaire.* The responses to the third questionnaire can be summarized by tallying the final vote and incorporating additional comments into the previous commentary.

Using the Results

Depending on the needs you are assessing, additional questionnaires may need to be developed and sent out to the respondents. The final questionnaire always should provide a prioritized list of items that can help in the planning process. The ranking of the items can indicate to the planners which items need to be addressed early in the planning process. When you have all the information you need, assemble the workgroup to review the data and develop a final report. This report should include a summary of all questionnaire results and recommendations for further planning based on the prioritization of the needs.

Reviewing an Example

An ad hoc Committee on Cancer in Women established by the American Cancer Society (ACS) decided to engage in a Delphi process to determine its future directions. All 14 members of the Committee agreed to be involved in the process, which was conducted over a three-month period. Three rounds of questionnaires were used, through which 22 issues were identified and then ranked using a scale from 1 (very high) to 5 (very low).

Each questionnaire iteration updated the participants about the results from their previous voting and the comments/suggestions offered for each topic. Additionally, in the third-round summary, the final average rankings were compared with the preliminary averages (from the initial questionnaire) for each topic so that the participants could note any trends over time. In this manner, the facilitators of the process provided the participants with helpful comparative information that could be incorporated into their decision making.

The top five (highest-ranked) topics were identified and used to guide the future actions of the Committee. The highest-ranked topic was to identify roles and strategies for the ACS to collaborate with other women's health groups and coalitions. Thus, over a relatively short period of time, the Committee was able to draw upon the written insights of its members to formulate directions for its future activity.

Online Resources

Visit http://healtheducation.jbpub.com/gilmore for links to these Web sites.

Community Advisory Committee of the Southern Health Board
An overview of methods for consumer and community participation in the planning of health services.

Delphi
Describes what a Delphi survey is and why it is used, and provides other related links on the Delphi process.
Results of the Delphi survey of disabled women.

Meeting the Needs of Women with Disabilities
Describes the characteristics of respondents on the Delphi survey.

Department of Agricultural and Food Economics
Describes an example of the Delphi survey in great detail including objectives, techniques, methods, and design.

Research and Training Center on Service and Coordination
Talks about focus groups and Delphi surveys.

Scottish Network for Chronic Pain Research
Discusses the Delphi Technique in pain research.

Western Rural Development Center
Outlines community assessment techniques. This site includes participant observation, social network analysis, the Delphi survey, the nominal group process, advisory groups, community forums, and application of these techniques.

References

Butler, L., and Howell, R. (1996). *Coping with Growth: Community Needs Assessment Techniques*. Washington State University: Western Regional Extension.

Delbecq, A., Van de Ven, A., and Gustafson, D. (1986). *Group Techniques for Program Planning: A Guide to Nominal Group and Delphi Processes*. Middleton, WI: Green Briar Press.

Gilmore, G. (1977). Needs Assessment Processes for Community Health Education. *International Journal of Health Education, 20,* 164–173.

Green, L., and Kreuter, M. (1999). *Health Promotion Planning: An Educational and Ecological Approach*. Mountain View, CA: Mayfield Publishing.

Moore, C. (1987). *Group Techniques for Idea Building*. Newbury Park, CA: Sage Publications.

Turoff, M., and Hiltz, S. (1996). Computer Based Delphi Processes. In Adler, M., and Ziglio, E. (Eds.). *Gazing into the Oracle: The Delphi Method and Its Application to Social Policy and Public Health*. London: Kingsley Publishers.

Interviewing

Introduction

If you like conversation, interviewing can be an exhilarating experience and an effective way to assess needs. Talking with people about their health needs, using the best interviewing techniques, is often as satisfying as planning a program to meet those needs.

Interviews can also bring good results. Compared to surveys, which are a very common and perhaps overused strategy for assessing needs, interviews are a more novel approach. People may resist completing one more questionnaire or refuse to participate in one more telephone survey. They may agree to an interview, however, because it is different. Most people like to talk about themselves. They feel flattered when selected to answer important questions and may be primed to give you good information.

At the same time, conducting interviews is not easy. The people you want to interview are often busy and difficult to contact to schedule an interview. When you do finally reach them, they may hesitate to interrupt their activities to participate. If they do participate, they may resist talking about their health.

Despite these difficulties, interviews are a good way to assess needs. If you have the time and other resources to conduct them, they can yield important information to use in planning educational programs.

Telephone and face-to-face surveys, discussed in Chapter 3, are a form of interviewing that follows a prescribed structure. This chapter focuses on some less structured interviewing approaches, which offer more flexibility and place more responsibility on the interviewer.

What do we mean by interviewing? A good interview is an exchange of information between two people: an interviewer and an interviewee. It may also include emotional expression and persuasion, similar to a good conversation (Gorden, 1998, p. 2). These characteristics are what make interviewing so fascinating. We obtain information from the interviewees, but learn about their attitudes and emotions as well.

74

Interviews can be either formal or informal. Informal interviewing is difficult to distinguish from ordinary conversation. The interviewer attempts to engage people in conversations, for example, about health-related issues. The conversation may occur in a very informal setting and usually is not arranged in advance. In some instances, the interviewee may not recognize this exchange of information as constituting an interview. Typically, the interviewer will know which questions to ask and will not refer to any notes or take any notes during the interview. As soon as possible thereafter, notes are written, typed, or dictated.

Although informal interviews can yield valuable insights, we will not consider them in this chapter. Because our focus is systematic needs assessment strategies, we will limit our discussion to formal interviews.

Reviewing the Strategy

Formal interviews are clearly identified as interviews. An individual is asked to participate in the interview. The interviewer states the purpose of the interview, describes how the person has been selected to participate, and explains that responses will be treated confidentially. During the interview, the interviewer will refer to an interview guide, usually called an interview schedule, and use some method of recording information.

Formal interviews are classified as highly scheduled, moderately scheduled, or nonscheduled (Stewart and Cash, 2003, pp. 88–90). At one extreme, a *highly scheduled interview* follows a very specific list of questions and instructions. For each participant, the interviewer must proceed through these questions in exactly the same way. Background information and instructions to the participant are read verbatim from a script. Follow-up questions to clarify the meaning of responses and instructions on recording responses are also clearly specified.

Highly scheduled interviews are conducted face-to-face or by telephone. They are practically identical to the face-to-face or telephone surveys discussed in Chapter 3 (Stewart and Cash, 2003, pp. 139, 158).

At the other extreme, a *nonscheduled interview* gives the interviewer much more freedom and responsibility. The goals of the interview are specified, but the interviewer must decide which questions to ask and in what order. The interviewer also decides how to summarize the information received.

A nonscheduled interview is not the same as the informal interview described earlier. Although the discussion may proceed in a relaxed, free-flowing, conversational manner, a nonscheduled interview is prearranged, has a stated purpose, and follows some type of overall structure. In these respects it differs from an informal interview.

A *moderately scheduled interview* falls between these two extremes. The interviewer follows a set of questions and suggested follow-up questions but is free to use them differently during the interviews. The wording of the questions can vary, as can the order in which they are asked. Additional follow-up questions are asked if the interviewer believes they would yield helpful information. He or she need not ask all questions of each participant if adequate answers to those questions have already been obtained. The interviewer receives some guidance about summarizing the information but must decide what to include and what to omit.

The word "schedule" can be confusing in this context. An *interview schedule* is a list of questions you plan to ask during the interview. It is easy to confuse this meaning of "schedule" (a noun) with the act of arranging a set time and place to conduct the interview (a verb). By a *scheduled interview,* we mean one that is conducted using a prepared list of questions; we do not mean one that is arranged in advance. A nonscheduled interview is one that does not use a prepared list of questions. This type of interviewing is different, however, from ordinary conversation that simply occurs spontaneously.

In this chapter, we will discuss only moderately scheduled and nonscheduled interviews conducted face-to-face. These interviews, which are sometimes called qualitative interviews, "sacrifice uniformity of questioning to achieve fuller development of information" (Weiss, 1994, p. 3). We will emphasize moderately scheduled interviews because they are more frequently used to assess health needs.

Advantages

Compared to highly scheduled interviews, moderately scheduled interviews have at least three advantages:

1. *They offer more opportunities to discover information.* A scheduled interview restricts the questions asked, so the information obtained is necessarily restricted as well. A moderately scheduled interview gives the interviewer freedom to explore certain subjects more extensively with some participants than with others. The interviewer may pursue a particularly insightful response in great depth and discover important information that had not been anticipated.

2. *They offer the opportunity to obtain more complete information.* The interviewer can ask as many follow-up questions as necessary to encourage participants to clarify and elaborate on their responses.

3. *They are especially well suited for obtaining valuable information from busy people.* If necessary, the interviewer can focus on the questions that each participant can answer most completely. By discussing in depth the areas they know best, the participants may feel they are using their time to best advantage. If pressed for time, the interviewer can skip other questions.

Disadvantages

Moderately scheduled interviews do, however, have some disadvantages compared to scheduled interviews:

1. *Interviewers need more in-depth understanding of the subject of the interviews.* Because the interviewers make more judgments during the interview about which questions to ask and which questions to omit, some knowledge of the subject is essential.
2. *Interviewers need more extensive training.* Knowledge of the subject is not sufficient by itself. The interviewers also need a more complete understanding of the purpose of the interviews and more opportunities to conduct and critique practice interviews. They also need to practice recording and summarizing the information.
3. *Data analysis is more difficult.* Information obtained from highly scheduled interviews primarily consists of quantitative data. By contrast, moderately scheduled interviews yield primarily narrative information. Analyzing the latter type of information requires making more judgments about organization and interpretation.
4. *Moderately scheduled interviews are more costly.* Typically, more time is needed to complete a moderately scheduled interview and record the information. More time is also necessary to train interviewers and analyze data. Because the interviewers need a background in health education, they may also cost more to employ than a typical survey assistant.

These advantages and disadvantages also apply to nonscheduled interviews—the difference is simply one of degree. Because nonscheduled interviews give even more freedom to, and place even more responsibility on, the interviewer, they offer even more opportunities for discovery and in-depth information. In turn, they require interviewers with more knowledge of the subject and more extensive training. Data analysis becomes even more difficult, and the whole process is even more costly.

When deciding how extensively to structure the interviews for assessing health needs, consider the following questions:

1. Do you want to measure what all of your participants know about certain healthy behaviors? Or do you want to discover what needs might exist? Generally, the more you want to discover needs, the less you should structure the interviews. For example, if you believe that poor diet and lack of exercise are major contributors to personal stress, you might use more structured interviews to determine what participants know about diet and exercise. If you are not predisposed to a diet-and-exercise focus, however, you might use less

structured interviews and discover other contributors to stress, such as financial difficulties, family conflicts, and various work-related pressures.

2. Do you have interviewers with a background in health? The less extensive their background, the more you should structure your interviews.

3. How much time and money do you have for this project? The less you have, the more you should structure your interviews.

Preparing for the Assessment

To prepare for interviews, follow the same basic steps discussed for surveys. Decide what you need to know, plan for Institutional Review Board (IRB) review and informed consent (Schiff, 2003), develop a budget, prepare your questions, test and modify these questions, develop a draft of an interview schedule or guide, conduct pilot interviews, develop data analysis procedures, and design the final schedule or guide. (See Chapter 3 for a more detailed discussion of these steps.)

How these steps are accomplished, however, is different for interviews. One difference relates to the development of questions. Although drafting, testing, and modifying questions is important, at least for moderately scheduled interviews, it is not as critical to develop the ultimate questions. Ultimately, the interviewers exercise some judgment over how questions are asked during the interview. They can clarify the meaning of questions if participants are confused.

A second difference relates to the development of an interview schedule or guide. Telephone and face-to-face surveys require a highly structured interview schedule. Moderately scheduled interviews, however, place more responsibility on the interviewer. They call for a list of questions to ask, along with suggested alternate wording and follow-up questions. With this kind of interview, the instructions need not be as specific nor the questions as precisely worded.

Nonscheduled interviews require even less structure. Typically, interviewer instructions include the goals of the interview and some guidelines to follow. The interviewers then proceed to ask the questions they believe will accomplish these goals. As the name implies, a nonscheduled interview does not even use a "schedule," but what is more properly called a guide.

A third difference relates to the development of coding and data analysis procedures. You should have some idea of how you plan to organize and analyze the data before you conduct the interviews. Try to anticipate the responses you are likely to receive and organize them into categories and general themes as best you can. This structure represents your best guess of how you will organize and eventually communicate the interview results. It will have considerably less detail than the coding and data analysis procedures developed for telephone and face-to-face surveys.

The structure is also more tentative. You can anticipate how you want to use the data, but you must always wait to actually receive the data before committing to a particular structure. The data may suggest other categories and themes that you could not anticipate before conducting the interviews. The less structured your interviews are, the less you can plan your coding and data analysis procedures in advance.

Moderately scheduled and nonscheduled interviews follow the same basic preparation steps as surveys, but less effort is required for some of them. Do not think you are getting off easy, though. The time you save preparing for the interviews you will spend—and more besides—after the interview.

Conducting the Assessment

Many steps used for conducting telephone and face-to-face surveys apply to moderately scheduled or nonscheduled interviews as well. You must select a sample of respondents to interview, recruit and train interviewers, and collect and record the data. How these steps are accomplished may vary considerably, depending on the interviews.

1. *Select a sample of respondents.* In some instances, the same probability sampling procedures used for surveys are appropriate for structured or nonstructured interviews. The less structured your interviews are, however, the more you may want to interview specific people. Remember that data analysis is a more extensive undertaking. Consider purposefully selecting a smaller number of key people, rather than drawing a systematic sample.

   You may decide to interview "knowledgeable insiders," known as key informants (Weiss, 1994, p. 20), who have the best perspective on the health needs of a particular community or organization. These individuals are selected because they can offer a broader view, for example, of community issues or societal trends than you would obtain from a random sample (Queeney, 1995, pp. 136–138). In such cases, you do not claim to have selected a representative sample of a given population. Instead, you purposefully select as many as 10 to 15 individuals who can offer critical insights.

   This approach of selecting a limited number of key informants is an example of a nonprobability or purposive sample, in which individuals are selected because they represent a range of diverse and important perspectives (Green and Lewis, 1986, p. 231).

   Be sure to include more people in your sample than you need to interview. Some individuals will decline to participate, and others will be virtually impossible to contact.

2. *Select and train the interviewers.* Because moderately scheduled and nonscheduled interviews place more responsibility on the interviewers, look for people who have both interviewing skills and a background in community health. Try to select individuals who are comfortable with and enjoy one-on-one, face-to-face situations. Look for people who are especially skilled in active and empathetic listening, people who can listen carefully to what interviewees are saying without preconceptions (Gorden, 1998, pp. 82–84). The more knowledge they have of the needs assessment project, the better. Knowledgeable interviewers have more credibility with interviewees and can make informed judgments about which follow-up questions to ask and which leads to follow.

Extensive interviewer training is necessary for moderately scheduled and nonscheduled interviews. As with telephone and face-to-face surveys, interviewers need to understand the purpose of the interviews, why they are important, and how the information will be used. They need instructions on contacting participants, handling ambiguous responses, and recording data. Compared to those conducting surveys, though, the interviewers need more information about the assumptions and philosophy that ground the project. They also need more instructions about what kinds of follow-up questions to ask. Finally, they need more opportunities to conduct and then critique practice interviews.

3. *Collect and record the data.* From your sample, develop a priority list of people to interview. Then begin to arrange appointments to conduct the interviews, preferably by telephoning or e-mailing the individuals. State the purpose of the interviews, which organization is conducting them, why they are important, and how the information will be used. Explain how the individuals were selected to participate and describe procedures for keeping responses confidential. Then ask for an interview at a time and place convenient for the participant. Specify how long the interview will take.

Scheduling the interviews can take considerable time. If you are using the telephone, you will not reach everyone on the first try. Attempt to determine the best time to call back, and try again. Some people will not respond to an e-mail request for an interview. Re-send your message after a few days, and then switch to the telephone to contact nonrespondents. Some people, particularly health professionals, are very busy and difficult to reach. Decide in advance how many "call backs" to make before skipping that person and contacting someone else.

If possible, conduct the interviews in places that have some association with your needs assessment. If interviewing health professionals about their needs for continuing education, offer to meet them in their offices or conference rooms. If interviewing consumers about their eating patterns, offer to interview them in their homes. These locations make participation in the interview convenient, but they also help the individuals focus on the subject of the interview. Be sure to arrive on time and conclude within the agreed-upon time.

When conducting interviews, take a few moments to set the stage. Although the participants have been contacted by phone to set up the interviews, they may have forgotten what was said or may not have listened very closely. Repeat the same information about the project to refresh their memories. Emphasize confidentiality. Have the interviewees sign a consent form that gives permission to use the information obtained (Seidman, 1998, pp. 56–58). If a telephone interview is being conducted, as with the telephone survey process in Chapter 3, respondents can respond verbally to consent-related questions, with notations made by the interviewer. A sample consent form is included at the end of this chapter.

The structure of an interview follows the same approach suggested for a survey in Chapter 3. Begin with questions that are relatively easy to answer. Ask potentially threatening questions near the middle of the interview, and hold demographic questions until near the end.

Interviewers should not refer to their interview schedule or guide as often as they would for a telephone or face-to-face survey. As much as possible, they should memorize the basic sequence of questions. Seidman (1998, pp. 63–78) urges interviewers to concentrate on the interviewees and take advantage of promising leads.

Remember that nonverbal cues are important for interviews. Gorden describes seven nonverbal behaviors that affect the quality of the data: physical distance, body position, touch, eye contact, facial expression, tone of voice, and pace of the interview (Gorden, 1998, pp. 67–74). Give the participants enough space to communicate with a sense of freedom, and position yourself to talk with them one-on-one as equals. Face the participants, and use your posture to communicate a sense of relaxed anticipation. Use good eye contact, nod, and smile appropriately. An appropriate tone of voice is also important. Some participants may respond to a soft-spoken, low-key interviewer. Other participants may need more lively prodding to reveal good information.

Probing techniques are an essential part of interviewing. Probing involves the use of neutral prompts to persuade interviewees to answer questions fully and completely. It is necessary when interviewees offer no response at all or give answers that are incomplete, irrelevant, poorly organized, or unclear.

Probes are used to gain greater detail, elaboration, or clarification. Who, what, when, where, or how questions can encourage interviewees to provide more detailed information. Gentle, approving nods and neutral comments ("yes," "uh-huh") or questions ("anything else?", "then what?") are examples of elaboration probes; they are designed to keep the interviewees talking. Silence is also an effective elaboration probe. Resist the temptation to fill in gaps in the conversation. Instead, let the interviewees do the talking as long as they have relevant information to offer.

To clarify ambiguous, unclear, contradictory, or irrelevant answers, ask neutral questions ("What do you mean?", "Why do you say that?"). You can also restate the original question, or summarize what has been said so far to encourage additional comments. Finally, appearing puzzled may result in clarification of a previous response. When probing, watch your emphasis on particular words, so as not to change the content or focus of a question.

Before concluding the interview, take a minute to review the schedule or guide to ensure that all pertinent questions have been asked. This review is especially important whenever questions have been asked in a different order from the schedule or guide, because it helps to prevent overlooking some questions. Finally, thank the interviewee for participating, and conclude the interview promptly.

Recording data poses special challenges for moderately scheduled or nonscheduled interviews. Unlike with surveys, writing every word in neat little boxes is not possible. Tape recording the interview is a possibility. A tape recording gives a complete record of the interview, which is important for some interviews. Some participants—particularly less educated people—may feel inhibited, however, by the presence of a tape recorder. More significantly, tape recordings require time and money to transcribe. Word-for-word transcriptions take from two to six hours for every hour of interview time (Gorden, 1987, p. 263).

Most needs assessments do not require the same precision in recording data as rigorous academic research. An alternative to word-for-word transcription is to summarize the interview. That is, one can transcribe critical statements in their entirety, but condense other statements. Repetitive and unimportant comments are skipped altogether. This summary will take significantly less time to transcribe, but it requires a knowledgeable transcriber who can judge what to include and what to omit.

For most needs assessments, effective note-taking during the interview is a good way to record data. This note-taking is more difficult than that performed for a survey. The questions are not as standardized, and the answers tend to be longer. The more structured the interview, the easier note-taking will be. When extensive note-taking is difficult during the interview, jot down key words or phrases. As soon as possible after the interview (preferably on the same day), expand these notes into a more detailed summary of the interview. Develop this summary on paper, at the computer, or on tape for later transcription.

Using the Results

What to do with the data is a critical problem when using moderately scheduled or nonscheduled interviews to assess needs. As noted earlier, talking with people about their needs can be exhilarating. After the interviews are over, however, you must make sense of the data stacked on your desk or stored in your computer.

With structured telephone or face-to-face surveys, this phase is more straightforward. The data collected from surveys are mostly quantitative, and procedures for analysis will have been developed during the preparation phase. Qualitative data typically are limited, both by the number of open-ended questions asked and by the scope of responses received.

In contrast, in moderately scheduled or nonscheduled interviews, the data are primarily qualitative. To some extent, you have tried to anticipate some responses and important categories during the preparation phase. Now you must determine whether these categories are still appropriate. Other categories may have become apparent during the interviews.

Use the questions asked during the interviews to suggest categories for data analysis. Remain open to other categories that emerge from responses of the participants. The more structured your interviews have been, the more appropriate your questions will remain for organizing the data.

The less structured your interviews, however, the more you will have to develop another way to organize the data. Look for themes that are suggested by one or more of the categories. This exercise may require reading interview notes several times, developing a tentative structure, and refining that structure over a period of time. Less structured interviews require less time to develop questions before the interviews take place, but they require more time and effort to organize and analyze data after the interviews are complete.

With moderately scheduled or nonscheduled interviews, you may not have asked everyone the same questions. Thus you cannot simply count how many participants expressed a certain need. Instead, you may have to present a narrative picture of the needs expressed. In this portrayal, use case examples from the best responses to illustrate the needs you are describing. The less structured your interviews, the more necessary this narrative picture. Seidman (1998, pp. 101–105) suggests constructing profiles or vignettes to illustrate the needs of particular individuals.

The concepts of reliability and validity do not directly apply to qualitative data, but the same underlying principles apply (Seidman, 1998, pp. 16–20).

Seek to establish the credibility of your data. Look for consistent responses within each interview as well as consistency across interviews. For example, if late in an interview a participant contradicts an earlier response, data from that interview are not as credible as data from an interview that is free of such contradictions.

Finally, consider how to present your findings to a planning committee or other interested groups. With a structured survey, you can rely heavily on a quantitative summary of the data and specific recommendations that follow. With moderately scheduled and nonscheduled interviews, however, more responsibility rests on you to present and interpret the findings in a way that is faithful to the data.

Reviewing an Example

Increasingly, interview procedures for needs and capacity assessments are being combined with other information collection procedures. A clear example of this more comprehensive approach is presented by Miller, Bedney, and Guenther-Grey (2003). They describe their efforts to assess the organizational capacity to offer HIV prevention services in a collaborative manner. Their seven-year, national multi-site (i.e., 13 communities), randomized trial primarily involved young men of color aged 15 to 25 who have sex with men. The overall prevention effort involved the promotion of safer sex behaviors. To build community capacity and sustain the prevention efforts, the project worked with community-based organizations (e.g., health departments, bars, entertainment promoters, youth groups, businesses, churches, civic organizations). To determine the long-term capacity of these types of organizations working in collaboration to offer the prevention intervention, a comprehensive Feasibility, Evaluation Ability, and Sustainability Assessment (FEASA) was developed. The three domains of the assessment process served as criteria for assessing organizational competencies.

FEASA, which used qualitative methods for data collection, included interviews, organizational records, and observations. For the interviews, rather than attempting to administer a uniform interview across all 13 sites, the investigators developed an "intents" guide to determine the most appropriate data collection procedures. The guide, derived from the project criteria, assisted the investigators in choosing the most appropriate information sources and assessment methods (e.g., observation, interviews, reviewing archival documents). Where used, the interviews involved key informants who were deemed to be knowledgeable of, or members of, the various target populations. During the pilot phase in the 13 communities, the investigators concluded that "FEASA has potential as a respectful and collaborative method for evaluating the capacity of community organizations to provide prevention services and act as research partners" (p. 595).

Online Resources

Visit http://healtheducation.jbpub.com/gilmore for links to these Web sites.

Community Advisory Committee of the Southern Health Board
An overview of methods for consumer and community participation in the planning of health services.

National Statistics Office
Republic of the Philippines notes of the National Demographic and Health Survey.

University of Surrey Social Research Update
Telephone methods for social surveys.

National Network for Child Care
An example of a student interview.

Health Bulletin
Role of the interviewer in data collection.

Palestinian Central Bureau of Statistics
An example of a health survey methodology, which includes various surveys and questionnaires.

Health Survey for England
Overview of a sample health survey done in England.

References

Gorden, R. L. (1998). *Basic Interviewing Skills.* Prospect Heights, IL: Waveland Press.

Gorden, R. L. (1987). *Interviewing: Strategy, Techniques, and Tactics.* Chicago: Dorsey Press.

Green, L. W., and Lewis, F. M. (1986). *Measurement and Evaluation in Health Education and Health Promotion.* Palo Alto, CA: Mayfield Publishing.

Miller, R., Bedney, B., and Guenther-Grey, C. (2003). Assessing Organizational Capacity to Deliver HIV Prevention Services Collaboratively: Tales from the Field. *Health Education and Behavior, 30,* 582–600.

Queeney, D. S. (1995). *Assessing Needs in Continuing Education: An Essential Tool for Quality Improvement.* San Francisco: Jossey-Bass Publishers.

Schiff, L. (2003). *Informed Consent: Information, Production, and Ideology.* Lanham, MD: Scarecrow Press, Inc.

Seidman, I. E. (1998). *Interviewing as Qualitative Research: A Guide for Researchers in Education and the Social Sciences,* 2nd ed. New York: Teachers College Press.

Stewart, C. J., and Cash, W. B., Jr. (2003). *Interviewing: Principles and Practices,* 10th ed. Boston: McGraw-Hill.

Weiss, R. S. (1994). *Learning from Strangers: The Art and Method of Qualitative Interview Studies.* New York: Free Press.

Informed Consent Area-Wide Telephone Worksite Survey

**Note: This informed consent form will be read verbally via telephone. Respondents will be required to state "I agree" or "I disagree" after each statement. The subjects' responses will be recorded by the telephone surveyor. Agreement with all five statements is required prior to the collection of any data.

1. I have been informed that the purpose of this study is to conduct an area-wide telephone survey, providing up-to-date statistics on smoke-free worksites in order to ensure the health and safety of employees and other community members.

I agree _____   I disagree _____

2. I have been informed that the survey will take approximately 15 minutes to complete.

I agree _____   I disagree _____

3. I have been informed that I am free to withdraw from the study at any time without penalty.

I agree _____   I disagree _____

4. I have been informed that the data will be held separately from the identification of the source. The County Health Department will retain names, addresses, and phone numbers of business participants in order to develop a list of smoke-free worksites, what smoke-free policies they have in place, when the policy was put in place, the status of current cessation support programs available to employees, and the level of interest in support services by the county. The survey results will not identify business finances nor health insurance information.

I agree_____   I disagree _____

5. I have been informed that the results of this survey may be published in scholarly journals without the mention of specific business names involved. The names of businesses that are smoke-free may be published in various media outlets as a way to positively recognize their contribution to the health enhancement of others.

I agree_____   I disagree _____

Recorder:

Name _____ Date _____

Signature _____

Source: Based on a consent form developed by Jill Hubbard, MPH candidate, and thesis committee, University of Wisconsin-La Crosse. Used with permission.

Assessments with Groups

There are many ways to conduct needs and capacity assessments with assembled groups. In the next five chapters, we will discuss the rather highly structured nominal group process and the less structured group assessment processes of focus groups, community forum, and participant observation. These strategies often are coupled with other assessment approaches in an effort to gain a more in-depth understanding of the reported needs and available resources. Additionally, we will address two important contexts for group needs assessments through technology and large-scale community-based formats.

6

Group Participation Process: Nominal Group

Introduction

The nominal group process was developed in 1968 by Andre Delbecq and Andrew Van de Ven (Delbecq, Van de Ven, and Gustafson, 1986) for assessments in business settings. It was based on the involvement of a few target audience representatives in a highly structured process to qualify and quantify specific needs. Since its development, the process has been used by a variety of professionals, including those in health care, human service agencies, voluntary organizations, university extensions, and educational settings (Moon, 1999; Queeney, 1995; Butler and Howell, 1993; Delbecq, Van de Ven, and Gustafson, 1986; Gilmore, 1977).

The nominal group process utilizes groups of five to seven people who have some knowledge of the issues being examined. Group members are asked to write responses to a question without discussing it among themselves. Each participant then shares one of his or her responses in a round-robin fashion, which continues until every response from each individual is recorded. The responses are clarified through discussion. Next, the participants select and rank a stated number of items that they think are the most important. The process may stop at this point, or discussion of the preliminary vote may be followed by a final vote.

Reviewing the Strategy

Although not a great deal of reading is required of the participants, possession of a clear and concise writing ability by the representatives greatly aids the process. Group involvement and understanding of health issues are important requirements of the representatives as well. The nominal group process provides both quantitative data, in the sense of voted-upon priorities, and qualitative data, in terms of a descriptive discussion of the problem (Delbecq, Van de Ven, and Gustafson, 1986). The qualitative data flow from the discussion is characteristic of most of the nominal group process. As part of this flow, members often provide critical incidents or personal anecdotes. The combined qualitative and quantitative data encourage professional reaction to client needs.

One difficulty that planners face when using the nominal group process is finding people who are willing to commit more than an hour of their time to the process. You may want to elicit participation by invitation—either of specific people or in an open situation in which people can reply with a commitment to participate. You also may seek cooperation from groups already in existence.

Advantages

Direct involvement of target groups. Those who may be most affected by a particular problem can be actively involved in its identification and scope.

Planned interactivity. There is an equal opportunity for all participants to share their ideas and be actively involved.

Diverse opinions. Because of the disciplined process, minority opinions and conflicting ideas are tolerated. The process attempts to avoid the evaluation of the ideas until the very end, when voting takes place. The process avoids arguments over semantics and wording through a clarification step.

Full participation. Because everyone is given an opportunity first to write down their ideas and then to discuss them, all are encouraged to participate. This higher degree of participation also tends to reduce the potential for control or use of hidden agendas by one or two participants.

Creative atmosphere. The nature of this group process, especially because it encourages writing down ideas and discussion, generates a creative tension and stimulates more ideas.

Recognition of common ground. Participants can discover areas of "common ground" among those who are present in the process, thereby enhancing the esprit de corps (Hair and Walsh-Bowers, 1992).

Disadvantages

Time commitment. Because of the amount of time required, there may be scheduling problems or difficulty finding participants who are willing to commit more than an hour of their time.

Competing issues. The group responses may deviate from the intended direction of the written questions, and participants may end up focusing on an issue different from the original.

Participant bias. Biases can enter into this process because it encourages sharing personal opinions, beliefs, and experiences.

Segmented planning involvement. Often the people who identify the need have no further involvement in the continuing program planning process.

Preparing for the Assessment

Four to eight weeks before conducting the nominal group process, you should complete extensive preliminary work.

1. *Identify potential groups for participation.* Ask yourself which specific populations make up your target audience during a particular programmatic phase or time period (for example, health education for primary prevention through immunizations). Next, consider what size of a sample of the target audience would reflect that group's needs, and identify specific people who can make up that sample and hence should be invited to a nominal group meeting.

2. *Enlist and train facilitators.* Attempt to have a facilitator for each grouping of five to seven people. Explain to the facilitators the purpose of the nominal group process and the specific steps they will be following. Also, have them assist you in the development of the question to be posed to the representatives.

   To fully prepare facilitators for the various details related to the process, we recommend taking them through a trial run as participants. Compose a question and then move the facilitators through the entire process. Following this experience, allow time for specific questions about the process. Emphasize the need for preplanning, particularly in regard to arrangement of facilities and materials.

3. *Develop the question.* This question must be clear and simply stated. Delbecq et al. (1986) have emphasized that the question should be generated after considering (1) the objective of the meeting, (2) an example of the type of items sought, (3) the development of alternative questions, and (4) the pilot testing of alternative questions with a sample group. A planning committee can be very helpful during this part of the process. One example of a question is, "What do you consider to be the major health problems you are facing at this time?" This type of question can be placed at the top of a sheet of paper and copied to hand out to the participants.

4. *Arrange for the facilities and necessary materials.* Consider where to hold a meeting of your representatives. You may find that it is best to hold several meetings at different locations for the convenience of the target audience. We have used this approach in multi-county assessments, for example. The following materials will be needed: one chalkboard, a flipchart (or other large writing surface for each small group), index cards (10 to 18 cards per person), handouts stating the group questions, pencils, and an information sheet to collect demographic data. The facilities you need include a large meeting room with enough space to accommodate smaller groups of five to seven people. The rooms should be equipped with tables or desks and

should be comfortable. If it is necessary to use the large room for several smaller groups, try to keep the groups as separate as possible so the work of one group does not influence or hinder other groups.

Conducting the Assessment

Using the nominal group process, follow these steps to conduct the assessment.

1. *Convene as a large group.* Explain the purpose of the meeting and the process that will be used. Establish a comfortable environment.
2. *Arrange the participants into groups of five to seven members, and assign a facilitator to each group.* Those selected as participants should be representative of, and knowledgeable about, the community in question. The facilitator should introduce himself or herself and emphasize the need for full participation. It is important to keep in mind that the nominal group process is designed to encourage everyone to participate openly without being impeded or overwhelmed by the titles of others in the group. (We have found it helpful for the participants to introduce themselves *without* stating their positions of employment.)
3. *Pose a single question to the group and have the participants write down their responses.* It is best if the question can appear in writing on a chalkboard or flipchart, and handout sheets. We have found that handouts are the easiest for the participants to use because they keep the question in front of the group members and provide space to write responses. Handouts also tend to keep the participants focused on the task, rather than gazing about the room. An alternative approach is to just write the question on a chalkboard, flipchart, or overhead projector transparency.

   Although the actual amount of time necessary to write the responses will vary depending on the particular question, an approximate amount of time would be 15 minutes. It is important that the group proceed in absolute silence. Such an approach enables each member to reflect carefully upon his or her own ideas, to be motivated by the observance of others who are working diligently by writing down their responses, and to be involved in a competition-free atmosphere where premature decisions do not have to be made.
4. *Elicit individual responses in a round-robin fashion.* One participant begins by giving a single response, the next gives a single response, and this process continues until each participant has contributed a single response. As the responses are stated, the group leader writes them on the chalkboard or flipchart, numbering each item. The same process is repeated until all contributions have been recorded. This

procedure enables each group member to fully participate. During this time, no discussion is permitted regarding the form, format, or meaning of a participant's response.

5. *Clarify the meaning of the responses.* Take time to be certain each response is clearly understood. Allow participants time to discuss what they meant by a particular response, the logic behind it, and its relative importance. However, this is not the time for argumentation and lobbying. The group leader must direct the proceedings so that only clarification takes place. Combine items with the same meaning.

6. *Conduct and discuss a preliminary vote.* From the original listing of responses, participants are directed to select and rank a stated number of items that they consider the most important. This ranking is accomplished by writing each one of the statements on a separate index card, and then rank ordering them. Make sure to distribute to each participant the appropriate number of index cards in accordance with the number of statements to be ranked. Delbecq et al. (1986) point out that group members can prioritize only five to nine items with some degree of reliability. Participants are asked to list one statement per index card. This is done by citing the statement number in the upper-left portion of the card, with a brief notation of key words from the statement in the center of the card. When all participants have accomplished this task for the statements they have selected, they should be encouraged to focus on the cards for ranking purposes. This will assist in decreasing any interference with their concentration during this important phase. Participants rank the cards by placing the rank number in the lower-right portion of the card and circling or underlining it. We have found that it is easiest to have individuals use a *reverse rank order* process. For example, if five items are being ranked, have participants list the highest-ranked item as 5 (i.e., the weighted value of the first ranked item). This will assist the facilitator as he or she lists the values on the chalkboard or flipchart during the feedback phase (see below). Otherwise, the facilitator must translate the actual rank values into weighted values prior to writing them on the board.

On the chalkboard (or flipchart), the group leader then records the rankings assigned to the statement selected by each participant (or has each participant come to the board to record his or her rankings). The facilitator totals the votes after all participants have contributed their rankings. The item with the largest numerical total represents the top-priority issue.

Discuss the various explanations related to the voting patterns. It may be valuable to discuss the high vote getters and the low vote getters. It also may be useful to redefine the meaning of selected items to be certain that all participants are clear on their meaning. Should any overriding concerns about the end result arise, it would be of value to provide the participants with another opportunity to vote.

7. *Conduct a final vote.* For this step, two procedures can be used: (1) as in the preliminary vote, select a stated number of the most important items and then reverse rank order them; or (2) select a stated number of the most important items and then *rate* them. To rate them, if seven major items are selected, each one could be rated on a scale from 0 (not important) to 10 (very important). This procedure provides insight regarding the magnitude of differences between the major items.

8. *Calculate the total vote.* Remembering that several groups of representatives may be participating in this process, it is important to calculate a grand total vote. First, the items from all groups are arranged into similar categorical areas (as closely as possible), and then the numbers from the rank ordering or rating exercises are added together in each categorical area. For example, if three items from group 1, two items from group 2, and four items from group 3 relate to health problems with rodent infestation, the total value (from ranking or rating) is calculated for all nine items. The resulting value is then listed for the categorical need area of "health problems related to rodent infestation." As the total votes are calculated for each categorical area, it will be realized that they can be placed in descending order. The categorical area with the largest number is considered to be of the highest priority.

9. *Compile and prioritize the data.* Once the data are compiled for each group, the next task is to combine similar need areas and the ratings (see **Tables 1 and 2**). Similar specific needs from each group are assimilated into a combined need statement. Also, the individual ratings for each specific need are combined (see step 2 in Table 1). Finally, general need areas are established and aligned with a grouped rating value for each area (combined and general need areas). The quantitative analysis relates to the final rating values.

Needs assessed through the nominal group process are carefully reviewed by the planning committee. While the qualitative and quantitative data presented in Table 2 appear quite absolute, one should not be guided solely by this tabular arrangement. Consider the commentary of your planning committee regarding additional needs that may not have been directly stated, but rather were implied. Consider potential reformulations of the general and combined need areas, as well as potential resources and barriers in addressing each one of the identified needs. Then have the planning committee establish the final priority listing.

TABLE 1
Nominal Group Process: Organizing and Combining the Data

1. Plot group results (for given geographical area).

Group I		Group II		Group III	
Specific Need	Rating	Specific Need	Rating	Specific Need	Rating
A	40	A	2	A	28
B	33	B	15	B	7
C	0	C	17	C	19
D	50	D	28	D	44
E	2	E	48	E	12
F	19	F	41	F	22
G	21	G	3	G	37
H	33	H	0	H	18
I	5	I	29		
J	16	J	35		
		K	21		
		L	38		
		M	9		

Note: These are *specific* need priorities.

2. Combine *similar specific* needs and their ratings.

Example: Item D (Group I) + Item F (Group II) + Item H (Group III) =

	Specific Need	Rating
	Combined need statement	109

TABLE 2
Nominal Group Process: Establishing General Need Areas

Final Ranking	Final Rating
1. General need area no. 1	221
a. Combined need statement	109
b. Specific need statement	44
c. Specific need statement	35
d. Specific need statement	33
2. General need area no. 2 (Follow same procedure)	

Note: May have to use "miscellaneous" and "unclassifiable" categories as general need areas.

Using the Results

One particular advantage resulting from the nominal group data compilation is that you have a quantified summary of the group discussion. This summary can be used in your planning process as one source of information. However, make certain to remind your planning committee that it is not to be construed as the end result of an explicit research process but rather as the summary of a group interaction process. Inform them that the numbers are not absolutes. Whether you choose to address those needs with the highest-priority listing will depend on multiple factors, such as lead time, available resources, target audience readiness, and opportunities for success. For example, you initially may wish to address a lower-priority need because of the availability of resources and the high chances for success. Where and when you start can be a planning committee decision.

Reviewing an Example

Moon (1999), a family physician, has described an interesting approach toward using the nominal group process with a small group practice engaged in family medicine. Titling his approach "Finding Diamonds in the Trenches with the Nominal Group Process," Moon focused on helping his practice look for ways to improve patient care and service by engaging the entire staff, rather than just the physicians. He noted that those "serving deep in the trenches of medical practice may actually have priceless ideas that no one has bothered to discover" (p. 49). Additionally, he found that involving more individuals in the nominal group process leads to greater buy-in for the next steps that need to be taken.

Two questions were used to focus the activity and stimulate suggestions by Moon's staff:

- What are five ways we could improve our current level of customer service?
- What are five things we should be doing to make our practice stand out?

The top response to the first question related to working as a team and helping one another in any way possible. It was noted that team building could be enhanced through cross-training, along with selected staff members updating others about their job responsibilities at staff meetings. The number one response to the second question was to have the providers telephone patients with any significant test results. This approach would provide timely feedback by the individual most able to provide the necessary information related to the results.

The nominal group process enabled those involved in the process to feel that their ideas were valued, along with receiving a summary of their top-ranked responses for immediate incorporation into their professional activities.

Online Resources

Visit http://healtheducation.jbpub.com/gilmore for links to these Web sites.

Community Advisory Committee of the Southern Health Board
An overview of methods for consumer and community participation in the planning of health services.

Michigan State University Extension
Outlines the nominal group process along with the advantages of using the process.

Center for Rural Studies, University of Vermont
Gives an overview of the nominal group process, the role of the facilitator, pros and cons of the process, and times to use the process.

Western Rural Development Center
Outlines community assessment techniques. This site includes participant observation, social network analysis, the Delphi survey, the nominal group process, advisory groups, community forums, and application of these techniques.

Designed to Involve
Provides an explanation of the nominal group process and lists resources for further reading on the process.

Virginia Institute of Government
Describes the nominal group process and outlines processes and steps of the technique.

Journal of Extension
Explains the nominal group process and its use as an alternative to brainstorming.

References

Butler, L., and Howell, R. (1993). *Coping with Growth: Community Needs Assessment Techniques.* Washington State University, Pullman: Western Regional Extension.

Delbecq, A., Van de Ven, A., and Gustafson, D. (1986). *Group Techniques for Program Planning: A Guide to Nominal Group and Delphi Processes.* Middletown, WI: Green Briar Press.

Gilmore, G. (1977). Needs Assessment Processes for Community Health Education. *International Journal of Health Education*, 20, 164–173.

Hair, H., and Walsh-Bowers, R. (1992). Promoting the Development of Assessment. *Journal of Community Psychology*, 20, 289–303.

Moon, R. (1999). Finding Diamonds in the Trenches with the Nominal Group Process. *Family Practice Management*, 6, 49–50.

Queeney, D. (1995). *Assessing Needs in Continuing Education: An Essential Tool for Quality Improvement*. San Francisco: Jossey-Bass Publishers.

7

Group Participation Process: Focus Group

Introduction

Focus group assessments are exploratory forms of qualitative research. One of the important purposes of these types of needs and capacity assessments is to engage in brainstorming and generate ideas (Edmunds, 1999). The focus group process has its roots in the group depth interview that was developed as a form of group therapy (Boyd, Westfall, and Starch, 1981). In the 1950s, this technique was borrowed from psychiatry and developed as a marketing research technique (Gage, 1980). It is in this area that the focus group gained prominence. Today it remains one of the most widely used marketing research techniques, but has expanded into other areas, including education, government, and social change and diversity arenas (Wycoff-Horn, Fetro, Drolet, and Russell, 2002; Edmunds, 1999; Schinke, Orlandi, Schilling, and Parms, 1992).

The focus group is typically an exploratory process that is used for generating hypotheses, uncovering attitudes and opinions, and acquiring and testing new ideas. It utilizes groups of 6 to 12 people that are fairly homogeneous in nature. The groups gather in a relaxed, informal setting to participate in an unstructured interview. A moderator has the task of focusing the group on the discussion topic and skillfully guiding the discussion in a way that stimulates interaction and encourages the sharing of feelings, attitudes, and ideas from all group members. With permission, usually the discussion is tape recorded and/or videotaped (Lacey, Manfredi, Balch, et al., 1993). If facilities are available, the focus group process can be viewed by administrative staff through a one-way mirror or via closed-circuit television. The focus group process aligns with the Social Diagnosis phase of the PRECEDE-PROCEED model (Green and Kreuter, 1999).

Reviewing the Strategy

Advantages

Low cost. The focus group is a relatively inexpensive method of using an exploratory approach to assess needs.

Convenience. It is easy to arrange and can be completed in a short amount of time (usually one and one-half hours). Because of the relative ease of implementation, a larger number of groups may be involved in this process than in other needs assessment strategies.

Creative atmosphere. The lack of rigid structure in the process encourages spontaneity and stimulates a wide range of ideas, emotions, attitudes, perceptions, and thoughts. A comment from one person may solicit ideas, feelings, or opinions from other people in the group. These comments are accepted as valuable information (Edmunds, 1999). The atmosphere is most important when sensitive issues are being addressed, such as the assessment of one's beliefs, attitudes, and perceptions about euthanasia (Wycoff-Horn, Fetro, Drolet, and Russell, 2002).

Ease of clarification. The focus group structure enables the moderator to obtain clarification if needed.

High flexibility potential. Unlike with the nominal group process, there is greater tolerance to deviate from the intended direction and to explore related ideas and concerns. Deviations are analyzed as carefully as other responses. However, it is the moderator's job to direct the group back to the topic if the discussion becomes irrelevant.

Disadvantages

Qualitative information. The data are exclusively qualitative, making coding, tabulating, and analyzing more difficult.

Limited representativeness. Sample sizes are quite small and randomization of the sample may be limited. Results are not easy to generalize (Schechter, Vanchieri, and Crofton, 1990).

Dependence on moderator skill. The results depend on the skill of the moderator. An inexperienced moderator or a moderator who has preconceived ideas can produce misleading results. Additionally, depending on how the meeting is conducted, some participants may not have an equal chance of participating. Some individuals may dominate the interaction, not allowing the more reserved individuals an opportunity to participate.

Preliminary insights. Because of the preliminary nature of the findings, as well as the focus on brainstorming rather than seeking consensus, the information obtained from focus groups usually does not stand alone. It is recommended that additional assessments that can add insight into the focus group findings be conducted before making any final decisions. A survey and/or nominal group process can serve this purpose very well.

Participant involvement. Recruitment of participants may be difficult, especially when trying to identify homogeneous groups in a short amount of time.

Preparing for the Assessment

Some market researchers have assembled a focus group within a few days. However, a little planning one to two months prior to the focus group discussion will help to keep the entire project on target.

1. *Develop an interview guide.* The interview guide outlines the scope of the need area that you will be assessing. Its purpose is to assist the moderator in introducing the topic or topics and focusing on these areas as needed throughout the discussion.

2. *Enlist a well-trained, experienced moderator.* The moderator is a crucial part of the focus group process. He or she must have good interpersonal communication skills and be able to quickly establish rapport and gain the confidence of the participants. Ideally, the moderator should fit in with the group. For example, if one is working mostly with women, the moderator should be a woman. This type of alignment is not always possible, especially when diverse groups are used. The same moderator should work with all groups. Familiarize the moderator with the goals and objectives of the needs assessment, as well as the mission, philosophy, and operations of your organization (if the moderator is from outside your organization). Make sure that you and the moderator become acquainted before beginning the focus group process.

3. *Determine the number and composition of the groups.* A good rule of thumb is to continue conducting focus groups until no new ideas are generated. A saturation point generally occurs after three or four groups. You may want to conduct more focus groups, depending on the kind of information you are seeking, the diversity of your groups, and time and cost allowances. If you want information from people of different backgrounds, you should identify those subgroups and conduct three to four focus groups for each subgroup. Do not rely on only one focus group (Lacey, Manfredi, Balch, et al., 1993).

   The makeup of the groups should be as homogeneous as possible. This consistency reduces variations in responses based on social, intellectual, lifestyle, or demographic differences. People from similar backgrounds are more likely to relate better to one another, and this composition will enhance the focus group discussion.

4. *Select participants.* Establish categories for participants based on criteria that will produce the most homogeneous groups. These categories may include gender, age, income, education, or other

demographic factors that may affect how people respond to the need area. For example, you may want to separate mothers who work outside the home from those who do not when assessing needs for health care services for children. The perceptions of these two groups may differ significantly and interfere with participants' abilities to relate to one another. Putting them together in one focus group may hinder the discussion.

Participants may be recruited from ads, lists, or other means using the quotas to screen the most appropriate candidates. They should have adequate background or experience so that they can contribute to the discussion. The participants should not know one another prior to the meeting, as their familiarity may influence group interaction. However, this recommendation is not always possible to achieve in small communities. In these situations, at least try to avoid placing close friends in the same group. The participants should not have taken part in a similar group interview for at least six months. Sometimes participants are paid for their involvement. Payment can be achieved in a variety of ways, such as monetary recognition of $5.00–$10.00, or social recognition of the participant's involvement in a worthy cause.

5. *Arrange the facilities.* Where the focus group is held has important implications for the success of the process. The setting should be very relaxed and informal. Sometimes it is appropriate to meet in the home of one of the participants. Avoid meeting around a large conference table, which is usually too large and formal to create a comfortable environment. The site of the focus group also may be influenced by what type of recording will be done. Use of a one-way mirror or closed-circuit television will require specific types of facilities, whereas tape recording or videotaping allows for more flexibility in choosing the meeting site. The most critical factors are that the room be comfortable to allow for open communications and that it be easily accessible to the participants.

Conducting the Assessment

1. Allow time for participants to gather and talk among themselves. This "fraternization" period gives them an opportunity to get to know one another and become more comfortable with the surroundings. The moderator should introduce himself or herself and then ask the participants to introduce themselves. Participants also can be asked to share with the group something about themselves that relates to the topic. For example, if the need area concerns children and you are meeting with young parents, you may want to ask them to tell the group something about their children.

2. The moderator then introduces the process and the topic. He or she should provide a brief description of the process and offer some guidelines for the discussion: Speak so that everyone can hear, speak one at a time, and be open and honest in expressing what you think and feel. The moderator can then make some general comments about the purpose of the meeting, being careful not to imply any expectations. Next, he or she makes a statement or asks a question that will open the discussion.

3. The moderator should carefully guide the discussion. Once the moderator initiates the discussion, group members are free to interact with one another in pursuing the topic. The moderator should take a less dominant role in the group, becoming involved only to ask questions that will keep the discussion moving, to introduce a new dimension to the topic, or to refocus the group if it has completely lost track of the topic. The moderator must carefully direct the discussion in a way that both maintains optimal freedom of the group interaction and elicits information that is relevant to the need area. For the moderator to focus on the group interaction, taping is strongly recommended. Trying to record notes about the event while it is happening will result in missed data. If only audio taping is available, the moderator may want to make some notations on behaviors throughout the interview.

4. If the process is being directly observed by other staff members through a one-way mirror or closed-circuit television, they should keep in mind several points. First, realize that what is being watched is work in progress. Second, listen actively and selectively, rather than for what you want to hear. Third, watch for nonverbal cues. Fourth, trust the moderator. If the process is not going well, however, let the moderator know. Seek participant permission for any recording.

5. Bring the discussion to a close. When all the areas outlined in the guide have been addressed, the discussion can be brought to an end. The moderator should ask the participants to offer a summary of what was discussed and what was resolved.

6. After several days, a follow-up call can be made to all participants to thank them for their involvement. At that time, you may ask for any additional information and ideas they may have generated since the focus group meeting took place.

The following list presents a summary of the key considerations for conducting a focus group (helpful as an overview to use in training others to assist in facilitation):

- The moderator should fit in well with the group. This person focuses the group on the discussion topic and guides the discussion so that interaction is stimulated and there is a sharing of ideas, feelings, and attitudes from all participants.

- Attempt to convene groups in which participants have similar backgrounds (within the group).
- Each group should consist of approximately 6 to 12 people.
- Have the groups gather in a relaxed, informal setting, and enable them to have time to "visit" briefly before getting started.
- At the start of the meeting, the moderator and participants should introduce themselves, and participants can be encouraged to make very brief comments related to the discussion topic.
- The moderator provides a brief introduction to the purpose of the meeting (e.g., to get participants' ideas about health-related issues and services related to families in a certain county) and offers discussion guidelines:

  1. Speak so that everyone can hear.
  2. Speak one at a time.
  3. Be open and honest in expressing what you think and feel.

- Ask the group members if they mind your use of a tape recorder so that you do not miss any important comments (you want to spend your time guiding the discussion, not writing too much).
- The moderator poses the questions and guides the discussion. The group members are free to interact with one another while making their responses. Remember, we are trying to get ideas, not achieve complete consensus.
- As a rule of thumb, continue the discussion on each question until no new ideas are being generated.
- Bring the discussion to a close by asking participants to summarize the key issues raised. You also can go around and have each participant offer one final comment.
- As soon as possible, prepare a summary of key ideas offered for each question.

Using the Results

Following each focus group, the moderator should meet with you to clarify what occurred in the session. A transcript should be created from the audio or videotape and then synthesized, analyzed, and interpreted. The information will usually be more significant if the people in the focus group become quickly involved without much prodding from the moderator, if the participants speak in the first person instead of the third person, and if they indicate some past experiences with this need area. Consider these points as you develop the report. The report should be written to include implications, interpretations, hypotheses, theories of how things are or could be, and recommendations. It should be integrated with quantitative and other qualitative data before making any decisions related to program planning. An example of this type of follow-up has been provided by Schinke et al. (1992), who conducted focus group assessments with Hispanic and African American adolescents in New York City. Following a series of seven focus group sessions held over a two-month time period, six expert panels of professionals were convened to corroborate the most reasonable educational recommendations for the prevention of HIV infection.

Reviewing an Example

One of the authors (GDG) conducted a series of focus group sessions in Vernon County, Wisconsin, while serving as the planning and evaluation consultant as part of a Family Preservation and Support (FPS) grant. To assess family health-related needs and resources across the three target groups of youths, adults, and older adults, members of the FPS Steering Committee were trained to serve as focus group facilitators. The basic principles for the process were outlined on a handout, which the facilitators used as a reference during the focus group sessions. A series of questions designed to elicit family health-related issues, as well as possibilities for individual and organizational resources that could be tapped (i.e., capacity building), were developed for each one of the three types of groups. An example of a health-related question for youths was as follows: "Generally, how has your family contributed to your current health and well-being?" An example of a capacity-building question for youths was as follows: "What kinds of contributions could you make to improve the quality of living in Vernon County?"

The process for each group throughout the county was dynamic. Individuals did not mind the use of a tape recorder because it was announced that people would not be identified, and that the tape recording enabled the leader to participate fully in facilitating the discussion. Indeed, some participants commented that today the use of some type of recording device during group discussions and interviews is quite commonplace.

The preliminary results indicated a wide range of family health issues and commentary on how society has changed today (e.g., it is harder for people to volunteer their time as they once did, given the need for many in the family to work outside of the home). Additionally, there were suggestions for individual and organizational contributions that could be made (e.g., setting up a "banking" process to record volunteer time contributions and responding in kind when the volunteers have special needs).

Online Resources

Visit http://healtheducation.jbpub.com/gilmore for links to these Web sites.

U.S. Department of Health and Human Services
Ways to manage focus groups effectively for maximum impact.

Community Advisory Committee of the Southern Health Board
An overview of methods for consumer and community participation in the planning of health services.

Research and Training Center on Service Coordination
Describes focus group methods and Delphi surveys.

Centers for Disease Control and Prevention
The CDC's Evaluation of HIV Prevention Programs using Qualitative Methods, which includes the Teacher's Focus Group Guide.

National Network for Child Care, Parents
An example focus group questionnaire for parents.

National Network for Child Care, Assessment
An example of a follow-up assessment of the focus group.

References

Boyd, H., Westfall, R., and Starch, S. (1981). *Marketing Research Text and Case Studies*. Homewood, IL: Richard D. Irwin.

Edmunds, H. (1999). *The Focus Group Research Handbook*. Chicago: NTC Business Books and the American Marketing Association.

Gage, T. (1980). Theories Differ on Use of Focus Group. *Advertising Age*, 51, 519–522.

Green, L., and Kreuter, M. (1999). *Health Promotion Planning: An Educational and Ecological Approach*. Mountain View, CA.: Mayfield Publishing.

Lacey, L., Manfredi, C., Balch, G., Warnecki, R., Allen, K., and Edwards, C. (1993). Social Support in Smoking Cessation among Black Women in Chicago Public Housing. *Public Health Reports*, 108, 387–394.

Schechter, C., Vanchieri, C., and Crofton, C. (1990). Evaluating Women's Attitudes and Perceptions in Developing Mammography Promotion Messages. *Public Health Reports*, 105, 253–257.

Schinke, S., Orlandi, M., Schilling, R., and Parms, C. (1992). Feasibility of Interactive Videodisc Technology to Teach Minority Youth about Preventing HIV Infection. *Public Health Reports*, 107, 323–330.

Wycoff-Horn, M., Fetro, J., Drolet, J., and Russell, R. (2002). Beliefs, Attitudes, and Perceptions of Selected Undergraduate Students about Euthanasia. *The Health Educator: Journal of Eta Sigma Gamma*, 34, 11–16.

8

Community-Based Needs and Capacity Assessment Processes

Introduction

Two very specific and popular group needs and capacity assessment strategies were addressed in Chapters 6 and 7. These assessments are typically used with groups that are formulated by the person(s) coordinating the assessment efforts. Complementing these assessments are community-based capacity assessments, which are conducted in natural community settings. The original work by Kretzmann and McKnight (1993), as described in Chapter 2, has been expanded through more in-depth descriptions of how to plan for and conduct capacity assessments (Kretzmann, McKnight, and Sheehan, 1997; Kretzmann, McKnight, and Puntenney, 1998; Dewar, 1997). It is important to point out that because of the clear distinction drawn by Kretzmann, McKnight, and Sheehan (1997) between needs and capacity assessments, these community-based approaches are specifically capacity assessments. Because they usually take place in distinct areas or settings in a community, these types of capacity assessments can be considered neighborhood capacity assessments. Capacity assessments provide an excellent opportunity for determining basic talents and resources that are imbued in the population (see **Figure 1**). They also represent a positive and productive way to meet and greet others in a neighborhood.

Complementing these types of survey and group discussion approaches for ascertaining individual talents and resources are several other community-based methods. The community forum (also referred to as a public hearing) is intended to address a focused issue in a community and to assess actual and perceived resources through a rather formal process. Additionally, participant observation affords the person(s) carrying out the assessment with a nonreactive group process. Importantly, one can think creatively in planning and conducting the community-based assessment processes so that reality is more fully reflected in the resulting information and insights.

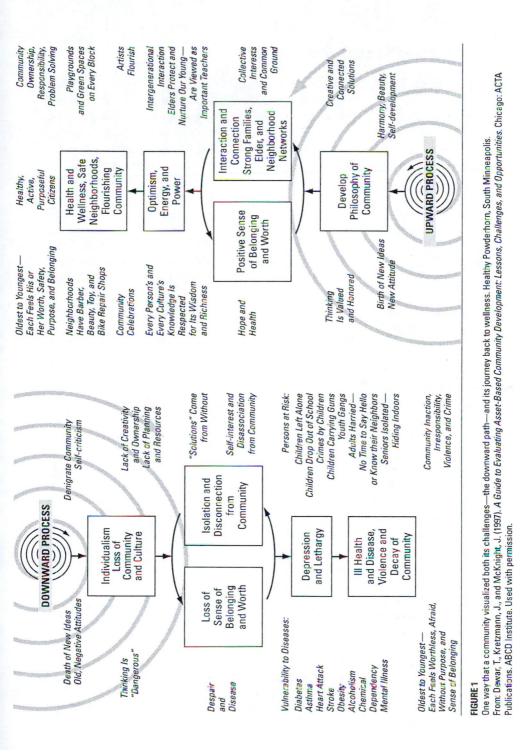

FIGURE 1

One way that a community visualized both its challenges—the downward path—and its journey back to wellness. Healthy Powderhorn, South Minneapolis.

From: Dewar, T., Kretzmann, J., and McKnight, J. (1997). *A Guide to Evaluating Asset-Based Community Development: Lessons, Challenges, and Opportunities.* Chicago: ACTA Publications. ABCD Institute. Used with permission.

Community Capacity Assessment

Reviewing the Strategy

Capacity assessments have their origins in Ivan Illich's Center for Intercultural Documentation in Cuernavaca, Mexico, in which educators participated in seminars to brainstorm creative educational models (Kretzmann, McKnight, and Puntenney, 1998). Drawing from this collective thinking and sharing approach, Denis Detzel brought back to Northwestern University the idea of developing a local capacity listing and referral service. This process, which soon became known as the Learning Exchange, had as one of its key goals the development of an "economical and efficient vehicle to collect, organize, and make accessible information about educational and recreational resources and opportunities in metropolitan Chicago" (Kretzmann, McKnight, and Puntenney, 1998, p. 3). A complementary goal addressed the encouragement of individuals "to assume the responsibility to teach, learn, and share their interests with others" (p. 3). Overall, the process of information gathering, storage, and retrieval stimulated an exchange of skills and talents, and fostered relationship building. Of note, the assessment process can range from simple to complex. An example of a simpler version of a community capacity survey is included in Appendix E.

Advantages

Can be simply developed and implemented. As long as the purpose of the assessment is clearly stipulated and followed by the planners, the capacity assessment procedures can incorporate a variety of information-gathering methods (e.g., brief survey, interviews, group discussions).

Provides opportunities for active involvement of residents. Individuals who reside in the neighborhood feel more engaged in the process and the value of the information derived. Additionally, because residents many times are involved in conducting the assessments, they have an added benefit of "meeting and greeting" others.

Process can be repeated at various times. Because the assessment is considered to be for the benefit of the neighborhood, residents are often more inclined to allow and facilitate multiple requests for information. For the multiple assessment contacts to continue, it is important for the residents to receive ongoing updates regarding how the information is being used to better their circumstances.

Disadvantages

Possible surface assessment affording more breadth than depth. While it is possible to develop a capacity assessment process of any degree of complexity, because of the usual intent to engage residents in the process (see the discussion regarding participatory community-based research in Chapter 2), the assessments tend to be simpler in format. While this consideration does not detract from the value of the process, commitment over time on the part of those involved will be necessary to encourage continuing engagement in future aspects of the assessment.

Initially, residents may be skeptical and want anonymity. Today, more than ever, community members are being inundated with requests for their time, resources, and identity. The emergence of multiple means of contacting people (e.g., electronic, postal, face-to-face), has led to well-founded concerns about being taken advantage of and being the target of identity theft. Such concerns may lead individuals to be reticent about becoming involved initially. One means of addressing this concern is to make certain that key community leaders (formal and informal) are involved in the early and continuing phases of the project, and to ensure that the community is updated on the effort from its early stages throughout its implementation.

Preparing for the Assessment

Clear steps must be built into the planning phases. At the outset, it is essential to identify a core group of volunteers. Kretzmann, McKnight, and Puntenney (1998) point out that paid staff can always be added during the later planning phases, but initially identifying a core group of dedicated volunteers who have most of the following skills will be most advantageous: record-keeping, advertising, fundraising, writing, and graphic design. Importantly, this part of the preparation process also achieves a degree of buy-in.

The next steps include the development of a plan. The plan should have clearly stated goals (future directions) with aligned objectives (e.g., developing an appropriate contact system). Each objective is then addressed by specific strategies and timelines for achievement. Even though the assessment process is itself a type of formative evaluation process, it will be necessary to develop an evaluation system for the overall assessment effort. The evaluative commentary from volunteers and residents will be helpful in detecting the degree and type of accomplishment of the objectives.

Kretzmann, McKnight, and Puntenney (1998) carefully describe approaches to developing information systems that will be used in an ongoing manner in the community. Overall, they view the information-gathering process as an ongoing venture, rather than a single effort conducted at one point in time. They delineate several types of files that can be developed as a part of the information system: a master card file with basic background, skill/talent, and contact information for those who are retained in the system; teacher/learner cards for individuals to signify their particular desired role in the process; interest cards on which individuals can indicate their interests in joining others for various activities; and feedback cards, which can be used to provide input regarding activities undertaken and a brief evaluation of one's involvement. For purposes of brief assessment, inventories such as the one in Appendix E can be used.

Bartholomew, Parcel, Kok, and Gottlieb (2001) complement the capacity assessment steps by delineating an intervention-mapping approach for health promotion. This process has five key steps:

1. Creation of matrices of proximal program objectives based on the determinants of behavior and environmental conditions
2. Selection of theory-based intervention methods and practical strategies
3. Translation of methods into organized programs
4. Integration of adoption and implementation plans
5. Generation of an evaluation plan (p. 9)

Conducting the Assessment

At the outset, it is important to have a stated purpose for the assessment. Keep the purpose simple and understandable for those involved in the capacity assessment process. Also, refer to the purpose frequently as a guide while developing the process. Kretzmann, McKnight, and Sheehan (1997) caution against collecting too much information, or information without a purpose: "Too much information, especially if it is not clearly related to community-building goals often becomes cumbersome and awkward to use"; additionally, people can "get so focused on the collection of data about individual capacities that they forget their vision for how assets will be tapped and gifts and resources shared" (p. 65). Clearly, it is important to consider how the information will be used.

Wherever possible, involve community representatives in conducting the assessment. These individuals are known by the community, and thus they should be better able to access a cross section of the population.

In terms of the methods for collecting capacity information, Kretzmann, McKnight, and Sheehan detail the following key questions (1997, pp. 66–67):

- What is the most effective way to collect information from our residents, given the resources at our disposal?
- How many of our community residents do we want to interview?
- How will our interviewers be educated and trained in the capacity inventory approach and process?
- What will happen to the capacity information once it has been collected? Who will be responsible for analyzing and maintaining it, and making sure it is available to be used toward meeting the organization's goals?

Using the Results

Once the data are collected, it is important to become immersed in them. Kretzmann, McKnight, and Sheehan (1997) point out that during this phase, a computer can be of great help, "but it cannot *understand* individuals and capacities" (p. 71). Thus, it is imperative that the compiled information be reviewed by a planning or advisory committee so that the various skills, gifts, talents, and interests of the assessed neighborhoods and communities can be categorized and aligned with the planned community-building efforts. Businesses also can be assessed regarding their capacities, and these resources can be aligned with the assessed individual gifts and talents (Kretzmann and McKnight, 1997). Overall, all of the assessed capacity information can be input into a data system for retrieval on an as-needed basis.

Community Forum

Reviewing the Strategy

The community forum, or public hearing, assessment approach is an attempt to identify needs and capacities of communities and neighborhoods through public meetings. While the main effort is to inform the public, these meetings also can seek the needs and capacity-related *insights* of those in attendance, usually at minimal cost (Butler and Howell, 1993). Witkin (1984, p. 130) notes that a variety of formats can be used in the community forum:

- Hearings enabling people to speak as long as they desire, an approach typically employed during more formal and official hearings
- Meetings in which each speaker has a limitation on the amount of speaking time
- Meetings that use a group survey, asking participants to rank or rate statements or respond to questions
- The small group approach, in which participants are divided into small groups for discussion and eventual feedback to the total group

Typically, the community forum approach is used to identify general areas of need and capacity, which are subsequently refined through additional strategies.

A community forum is a public meeting that invites participation from anyone in the community wishing to offer his or her perspective on a particular issue. It seeks to involve a broad cross section of the community in an effort to review various points of view. In some cases, a community forum is conducted by a unit of local government as a public hearing, following the statutes governing that unit. At other times, a community forum is conducted less formally.

Advantages

1. A community forum is relatively straightforward to conduct. People are invited to come to a community facility to express their views on

an issue, one at a time. You record what they say. Compared to a nominal group process, for example, a community forum is much simpler to run and requires fewer staff members with less extensive training.

2. A community forum is relatively inexpensive. The only costs are for publicity, staff time to attend the forum, staff time to record and analyze the information gathered from the forum, and possibly rental fees for the facility used.

3. Because the forum is publicly advertised, it offers the opportunity to hear the views of all segments of the community.

4. People can participate on their own terms. They can come to the forum and simply state what is on their minds. They do not have to master a certain technique or follow a structured set of questions.

5. A community forum can help identify people from the community who are most interested in addressing the determined needs. The people who take the time to participate in a forum are likely to be those who feel most strongly about the issues and want to see them addressed. They are people who may later be involved in planning ways to meet the identified needs, thus enhancing the overall community capacity.

Disadvantages

1. It is often difficult to achieve good attendance. Although a forum usually has the potential to attract a cross section of the community, in reality it rarely does. As a result, the people who do participate will offer only a partial view of the needs that exist.

2. Participants in the community forum may tend to represent special interests. They have the most to gain or lose, so they usually are most highly motivated to come. People with less of an investment in the issue may have valuable insights to offer, but because they are not as highly motivated, they may not take the time to attend. Therefore, although the participants in a community forum may be good candidates for helping to meet the identified needs later on, they also may represent special interests that can skew the planning process.

3. The forum could degenerate into a gripe session. Because the format allows people to say what is on their minds, they may avoid focusing on particular needs to be addressed. While other strategies for needs and capacity assessment can be more difficult for the participants to relate to, they do introduce some structure that can prevent the process from evolving into an unending series of complaints.

4. Data analysis can be time-consuming. Because the information gathered from a community forum may not follow any particular pattern, it will be necessary to develop a structure after the forum and determine the best way of summarizing and presenting the findings.

The best way to consider the role of a community forum in the needs assessment process is as a test of needs that have been identified through some other process. Previously identified needs can be presented to the public through the forum to determine whether the public confirms them as needs. It is a way of legitimizing needs that have already been suggested as well as allowing new needs to surface.

Preparing for the Assessment

1. *Develop one or more questions that the forum will address.* It is better to use questions rather than present a general topic, as the participants will have an opportunity to focus their comments. The question orientation also makes it easier for them to respond, and may increase their motivation to participate.

2. *Determine how many forums to schedule.* There are several criteria to keep in mind when determining how many forums to conduct. If you want to obtain the broadest possible participation, you may need to schedule several forums at different times and in different places. If you want to draw people from a wide geographical area, then you will want to schedule them so as to minimize travel distances. Keep in mind the type of people you want to attend. An evening forum usually will be necessary to attract working people, but its timing may discourage elderly people from attending; they may need an opportunity to attend a forum during the day. A final criterion is the amount of time and money you have to complete your needs and capacity assessment. Although a community forum is relatively inexpensive, each forum does involve certain costs.

3. *Schedule the forum or forums in accessible places.* Often a well-known public facility located in a convenient location (e.g., a public library, city hall, local school, or community center) works well. Even hospitals and colleges can be used if they are known for their community service work. When scheduling the facility, consider the availability of parking at the time the forum will be held.

4. *Publicize the forum widely.* Take advantage of as much free publicity as possible from the mass media. Send press releases to local daily and weekly newspapers, radio stations, and television stations. Follow up these news releases by contacting news reporters. Try to arrange an appointment to discuss the importance of the upcoming forum and encourage the release of an article in advance of the forum. Try to arrange to be interviewed by radio and television reporters, and participate in call-in talk shows or local community features if possible.

Do not rely solely on the mass media, however, to publicize the forum. Consider mailing flyers to organizations interested in the issues to be addressed, and ask these organizations to publicize the forum to their members (perhaps by placing an announcement in their newsletters). Place notices in widely used public sites, such as public libraries, banks, restaurants, and supermarkets. If your budget permits, you may want to mail letters or flyers directly to individuals or groups you especially want to attract to the forum.

In the publicity materials for the forum, make sure to specify what participants will be asked to do. Clearly identify the question or questions they should address. Give them the opportunity to speak at the forum and/or to submit written commentary if desired.

5. *Make the necessary on-site arrangements.* Make sure enough chairs are available. Typically, the staff would be seated at a table slightly removed from the participants, with paper and pens to take notes as desired. If the room is large, microphones should be provided both for the participants and for the staff members who may wish to ask questions. A staff member should register the participants as they arrive and receive any written materials they wish to submit. Be sure the room is well marked both outside and inside the building. If the budget permits, providing light refreshments can contribute to a congenial gathering.

Conducting the Assessment

1. *Start the forum on time.* The person conducting the forum should welcome the participants, thank them for coming, introduce himself or herself and the other staff members, briefly state the purpose of the forum, and explain how the event will be conducted.

2. *Keep the forum moving.* Invite the participants to participate in the order in which they registered upon arrival, unless you have in mind some other plan for the order of presenting comments. Encourage the participants to keep their remarks within the allotted time, typically five or ten minutes. After the participant comments, allow each staff member present to ask the participant any questions for clarification or follow-up. Usually, you will not want to have your staff or members of the audience engage in a discussion of what was said. The purpose of a forum is to allow everyone an opportunity to speak in an orderly fashion, with opportunities for clarification by staff members.

3. *Conclude the forum when appropriate.* It is difficult to predict what will happen during a community forum. If only a few people show up, there will be more opportunity to ask questions of the participants. If a large crowd attends, it may be best to restrict the follow-up questions to keep the forum from dragging on too long. Thank the people for their participation and assure them that their commentary

will be used in planning to address the needs identified. You may also want to remind them that some may be called upon in the future for program development involvement.

Using the Results

As noted earlier, it is difficult to structure the data analysis until after the forum is complete. Analyzing the data from a community forum can be similar to analyzing the data from key informant interviews, as explained in Chapter 5. Read through the information to see what categories emerge and then summarize the data under each of those categories. Again, a community forum may be best used to confirm needs determined by other needs assessment strategies. Compare the needs that surfaced from the forum with these other needs before making final decisions about which ones should be addressed.

Participant Observation

Reviewing the Strategy

Health professionals sometimes place themselves in group situations for varying amounts of time in an effort to gain a sense of group health needs and available resources. Examples include attending a community group's series of meetings as a known representative of a health agency without serving in any official capacity and attending such meetings as a concerned citizen with one's professional responsibilities undeclared. In both cases, the health professional attempts to accumulate visual and auditory cues, which eventually may lead to clear patterns of an expressed need and opportunities for group contributions. No matter how well integrated into the group this person becomes, however, an inherent bias may be interjected into the group discussions and interactions due to his or her presence (Webb, et al., 1966, p. 113).

Advantages

1. Participant observation enables one to observe the unique interaction of group members directly, rather than serving necessarily as an outside observer.
2. Typically, there is minimal outside interference (e.g., activities of other groups) as one views the selected group members working together in their natural environment.
3. Observation at a series of group meetings is possible. This flexibility provides several opportunities to examine trends over time, and, if necessary, have them clarified and corroborated by certain group members.

4. There is flexibility in the information-gathering procedures so that one does not feel "locked in" to a single process during one event.

Disadvantages

1. The observer may potentially exert (knowingly and unknowingly) some influence on the discussion patterns and decisions, and there is observer inclination to pick up on only certain types of information (Webb and Weick, 1983).
2. Participant observation is a time-consuming activity. In addition to the time spent sitting through an entire meeting, you have to allow travel time to and from the meetings, and time (very soon after the meeting) to commit your observations to writing.
3. Attendance at more than one meeting of the group is usually necessary. Unlike a nominal group process or a community forum, both of which are very structured group meetings designed to yield very specific information on one occasion, participant observation is much more unpredictable and open-ended. Although one meeting can yield much information about health-related needs and potential resources, the next two or three meetings may provide little information. Due to the time and staff resources that must be committed to such a venture, you should determine whether the benefits will be worth the cost.

Preparing for the Assessment

1. *Determine specifically what you are looking for.* If you want to try to answer very specific questions about health-related needs from observing a group, be very focused in your observations. Pay particular attention to those group interactions that help answer those questions. More often, however, you may not have such a sharply focused list of questions. In that case, you will want to pay attention to a wider range of group interactions. Also, determine the scope of your participant observation activities. Determine how many groups are to be observed, how many meetings of each group to attend, and how active you want your observers to be during these group meetings.
2. *Select your observers.* The participant observer may be you, or you may need additional observers if you plan to observe more than one group. More significantly, you may decide in some situations that you are not the best person to observe the group. Many of the group members may know you, and you may believe this relationship will unduly bias the group interaction. In those situations, it may be best for the observer to be someone they do not know. Also, your

professional status may hinder the group's willingness to contribute. If so, it may be advisable to recruit people who can more easily blend in with the group members. Just as good teaching is often considered an art, so is good participant observation. Some people are more naturally gifted in this area than others. Thus, in the observer selection process, consider whether individuals have the appropriate personality to become good observers and how much experience they have had working with groups.

3. *Train the observers.* Explain the purpose of the observation to your observers and tell them what to look for. Discuss good techniques of group observation (see "Conducting the Assessment"). Develop handouts describing how to use these techniques in more detail, and arrange opportunities to discuss these observations. Also, discuss how to record observations and provide opportunities to practice and critique.

4. *Gain access to the group.* Obtain permission to attend group meetings. Explain as much as you can about your purpose in observing the group without undermining what you are trying to accomplish. You want to be honest about your intentions and do not want to deceive participants about your activities. Tell them what organization is conducting the assessment and how the data will be used. Assure the group members that the data will be kept confidential. In some cases, it may be best to have the group members sign a statement of permission to participate in your process.

Conducting the Assessment

1. *Be as inconspicuous as possible, but try to position yourself so that you can observe the group members.* Facial gestures are an important part of any group observation. If your role is strictly to observe, you may be able to sit off to the side. If you are going to participate in a limited way, however, you will need to be more a part of the group.

2. *Limit recording of data during the meeting as much as possible.* One of the best ways to record data is to take limited notes during the meeting by using a small notepad to jot down key phrases and impressions you want to remember. Keep the note-taking as inconspicuous as possible. If the group members see you writing down every word they say, they may not feel as free to share what they really have in mind.

3. *Using the notes taken during the meeting as a guide, develop extensive descriptions of the meeting as soon as possible after the meeting ends.* If you have been able to focus your observation on some key

issues, describe what happened that is relevant to these issues. If your observation is not as focused, then you will have to describe the meeting in greater detail. These field notes can be dictated for later transcription. (Remember that this dictation will increase the cost of your observations, because someone will have to transcribe it later.) If possible, develop these field notes right after the meeting. Even with no notes available, you will be surprised how much you recall from the meeting and how extensive your eventual field notes will be.

4. *Critique your observations between group meetings.* The day after the meeting, take time to reread your field notes and reflect on what you have observed. Ask yourself what you are learning and whether you are observing the right things. This self-critique will help you be more focused for the next meeting. If you started participant observation without a truly specific focus, you should find that you can become more focused with each meeting observed. If more than one person is observing groups, it may be helpful to have them periodically meet to share notes. What one person is observing may be confirmed by another observer's experience. Also, this collaboration may assist the other observer to have a better idea of what to look for at the next group meeting.

Using the Results

Analysis of the data from participant observations is similar to the analytical method used for interviews. If you have specific questions in mind that you want answered from the assessment, organize your findings around these major questions. If you do not have specific questions in mind, look for categories and then group the categories into themes. This latter approach is a more inductive process.

Trends emanating from the participant observation process can be aligned with the prioritized needs evolving from other needs assessment strategies. This additional information is incorporated into the decision-making process so that the next steps can be established. The decision-making process can be as straightforward as initiating planning committee discussions regarding what the prioritized needs are and then reviewing the pros and cons of the objectives and methods to address the needs.

Reviewing an Example

Dewar (1997) described the *Healthy Powderhorn Story,* which took place in south Minneapolis. One of the major efforts of this community-organizing initiative was to "uncover the resources and talents already existing in the community" (p. 15). An asset-based approach was taken to focus on community building. Importantly, the community had identified several challenges that needed to be addressed:

- How to mobilize the community and its assets around health action and cultural practices;
- How to deinstitutionalize community residents and their organizations in their approach to both individual and collective health;
- How to develop and run an effective community intermediary that is connected to, and truly respectful of, the values and aspirations of community residents; . . .
- How to document the impact, and report on progress toward goals in ways that would be credible, community sensitive, and doable (pp. 17–18).

Assessments of talents and resources emerged from discussions conducted at community meetings (during a 26-month period, 249 neighborhood meetings were held with structured listening opportunities serving as capacity assessments). Emerging from the suggestions were Community Health Action Teams (CHATS), which facilitated walking clubs, Native American spirituality classes, and the like.

Online Resources

Visit http://healtheducation.jbpub.com/gilmore for links to these Web sites.

Community Advisory Committee of the Southern Health Board
An overview of methods for consumer and community participation in the planning of health services.

Western Rural Development Center
Community assessment techniques. This site includes participant observation, social network analysis, the Delphi survey, the nominal group process, advisory groups, community forums, and application of these techniques.

Latino Needs Assessment Child Care Program
An example of a needs assessment.

U.S. Public Health Service
A report on community forums for youth violence and public health.

The Nature and Society Forum
A nonprofit community-based organization that promotes the health and well-being of individuals and the natural environment.

Women's Health Forum
Commissioned papers providing links to sessions and workshops.

References

Bartholomew, L., Parcel, G., Kok, G., and Gottlieb, N. (2001). *Intervention Mapping: Designing Theory and Evidenced-Based Health Promotion Programs.* Mountain View, CA: Mayfield Publishing.

Butler, L., and Howell, R. (1993). *Coping with Growth: Community Needs Assessment Techniques.* Pullman, WA: Washington State University, Western Regional Extension Service.

Dewar, T. (1997). *A Guide to Evaluating Asset-Based Community Development: Lessons, Challenges, and Opportunities.* Chicago: ACTA Publications.

Kretzmann, J., and McKnight, J. (1997). *A Guide to Mapping Local Business Assets and Mobilizing Local Business Capacities.* Chicago: ACTA Publications.

Kretzmann, J., and McKnight, J. (1993). *Building Communities from the Inside Out.* Chicago: ACTA Publications.

Kretzmann, J., McKnight, J., and Puntenney, D. (1998). *A Guide to Creating a Neighborhood Information Exchange: Building Communities by Connecting Local Skills and Knowledge.* Chicago: ACTA Publications.

Kretzmann, J., McKnight, J., and Sheehan, G. (1997). *A Guide to Capacity Inventories: Mobilizing the Community Skills of Local Residents.* Chicago: ACTA Publications.

Webb, E., Campbell, D., Schwartz, R., and Sechrest, L. (1966). *Unobtrusive Measures: Nonreactive Research in the Social Sciences.* Chicago: Rand McNally and Company.

Webb, E., and Weick, K. (1983). Unobtrusive Measures in Organizational Theory. In J. Van Maanen (Ed.), *Qualitative Methodology* (pp. 209–224). Beverly Hills, CA: Sage Publications.

Witkin, B. (1984). *Assessing Needs in Educational and Social Programs.* San Francisco: Jossey-Bass Publishers.

Technology-Supported Assessments

Introduction

Rapid technological change dominates our lives today. Advances in technology have led to many changes in health care and health promotion. Advances in communications technologies offer seemingly endless opportunities to change the ways we conduct business, use community services, and communicate with friends. Developing the Internet has led to a major revolution in our world. Concerns about linking rural areas electronically are beginning to be addressed in the United States as well as in other countries. As an example, Dutta, Jena, and Panda (1996) have described the use of assessments through distance education technology in India in an effort to develop strategies for health care delivery training.

This explosion in technology creates opportunities to assess needs and capacities in new ways, especially involving people located some distance from one another. Examples include audio, video, and computer conferencing. Equipment for these strategies is typically located in educational institutions, county courthouses, public libraries, medical facilities, and many corporations. Some conferences require specially equipped facilities, while others can use desktop computing equipment available at individual workstations.

Reviewing the Strategies

Audio Conferencing

Audio conferencing is perhaps the most basic use of technology to assess needs. Essentially it connects people by telephone. Sometimes a dedicated line is available to connect the participants, but more commonly the audio conference uses standard telephone lines. Newer telephones often have a conference call feature that enables the conference moderator to connect the participants directly. Alternatively, each participant might dial a central telephone bridge number and use a special code to connect to the conference.

A speaker phone with a mute button is highly recommended if at all possible to free the participants' hands for writing and shuffling papers and to ensure optimal audio quality. A speaker phone also enables participants to shift their posture and move around from time to time. With this arrangement, a productive audio conference can continue as long as an hour. After an hour, the conference may become difficult to sustain. If additional time is needed, schedule another conference call at a later time.

Audio conferencing can suffer from inappropriate acoustical conditions and the relatve lack of control over the order in which participants speak. It requires discipline on the part of the participants to pay close attention to who is speaking and what is said. An effective moderator is essential to help maintain control of the conference and to ensure that everyone has a chance to participate.

A variation of audio conferencing makes use of online computers. This type of computer-enhanced audio conferencing is sometimes called *audiographics*. Participants use a two-way audio conference connection and a "real-time" computer connection via a modem. The computer connection enables the conference moderator to send diagrams, charts, or other schematics. Computer graphics and prescanned images are "called up" on the screen when needed during the conference. Using special "writing pads" and pens, participants can respond to questions directly on the computer screen. What one person writes on the pad, everyone else sees simultaneously on the computer screen. Usually this audiographics system also involves the use of a slow-speed video camera for transmitting still images to each computer screen.

Advantages

1. *Very accessible.* Virtually everyone has a telephone. A conference call can bring together people who are widely scattered geographically.
2. *Comparatively inexpensive.* A local conference call has no direct costs. Although long-distance charges can mount for conference calls connecting several individuals, they are still less than costs for other technologies.
3. *Relatively quick process.* A typical conference call is shorter than a face-to-face meeting and does not require participants to travel.
4. *Encourages busy people to participate.* People who do not have time to travel out of town to attend an extended face-to-face meeting might agree to participate in a one-hour conference call.

Disadvantages

1. *Limited interaction.* A conference call offers verbal communication without the benefit of facial expression and other nonverbal cues.

2. *Requires people who are comfortable with verbal expression.* Participants are isolated from others on the line without the opportunity to observe expressions and receive encouragement from other people.

Computer Conferencing

The Internet has enabled people to connect through their personal computers to other people in various parts of the country and all over the world. Major advances in computer technology continue to expand the possibilities for information sharing at a rapid pace.

As more and more people have personal computers and Internet access both at work and at home, opportunities to assess needs using their computers become available. The key to a computer conference is having each participant connect to the Internet, either using a direct connection through work or a home subscription service.

Both synchronous and asynchronous computer conferences are possible. The simpler and more common approach is the asynchronous conference, which calls for participants to send and respond to messages during a prescribed period of time. This period may theoretically be as short as one hour but more likely will be as long as a week or even a month. During this period, participants agree to respond to questions, either directly by e-mail or through a listserv subscription.

In contrast, a synchronous computer conference requires all participants to be online with their computers at a prearranged time. Typically, a subscription service is used to set up a "chat room" or "instant messaging." Participants receive directions for logging onto their computers and gaining access to the discussion. They then proceed to converse with one another in written form using specified commands and directions. The dialogue that appears on the screen resembles a script for a dramatic production.

A variation on synchronous computer conferencing is the *webconference,* which combines computer conferencing with audio conferencing. Participants connect to the audio conference and then individually connect their computers to a preassigned Web address. PowerPoint slides or other visuals can be uploaded to a conference server and then discussed during the conference. The visual material can also include various interactive tools. People can participate anywhere they have access to the Internet and a phone, provided they have more than one phone line available.

Advantages

1. *Becoming more accessible.* Personal computers are now standard equipment in the workplace, and virtually all professionals have access to them. An increasing number of people have computers in their homes and access to the Internet as well.

2. *Comparatively inexpensive.* Once people have access to a personal computer, they will need an Internet connection at home or at their workplace. Assuming this basic equipment is available, most people will not incur any direct costs to participate in a computer conference. Although some people may incur long-distance telephone charges to connect to the Internet at home, most subscribers pay a flat monthly fee for unlimited Internet use.

3. *Relatively quick process.* The length of a synchronous computer conference is approximately the same as the length of an audio conference. An asynchronous computer conference could span a period of several weeks, but the actual time necessary for participants to read and respond to their messages is probably no more than 20 minutes at any one time.

4. *Encourages busy people to participate.* As with audio conferencing, people who are reluctant to participate in a face-to-face meeting might welcome the opportunity to join a computer conference.

5. *Novel approach.* Some people grow weary of having to attend one more meeting or participate in yet another conference call. For them a computer conference offers the opportunity to do something different, and their curiosity may overcome their initial resistance.

6. *Participants not influenced by socioeconomic status differences.* Because they cannot observe or talk with one another, participants do not pick up visual or verbal cues to socioeconomic status, unlike in face-to-face communications.

Disadvantages

1. *Limited interaction.* Computer conferencing involves responding in written form to other written information, unless it is combined with audio or video conferencing in some way.

2. *Requires people who enjoy written interaction.* Participants are isolated from one another and, unless combined with audio or video conferencing, cannot benefit from voice or facial interaction. As a result, computer conferencing is most useful for people who are comfortable using computers and enjoy written communication.

3. *Difficult to reach certain populations.* The proliferation of personal computers and the growing number of people with access to the Internet are making involvement of professionals in computer conferences quite realistic. For reaching a cross section of the general public, however, and especially lower-income, younger, or older populations, a computer conference is not as feasible.

Video Conferencing

Satellite technology has been used to offer credit courses and professional seminars for more than two decades. Unfortunately, this technology offers only one-way video and one-way audio communication from the instructors or speakers to the participants. To ask questions or offer comments, participants must initiate a telephone call on a separate line, typically to a toll-free number, or send an e-mail or facsimile message. This form of video conferencing is very expensive, requiring uplinking satellite equipment and a studio facility at the origination site and downlinking satellite equipment at each receive site. Current satellite technology is too expensive and too limited to use for needs assessment. Future developments may lead to widespread use of smaller and less expensive home satellite dishes, which may have potential needs assessment applications.

More promising than satellite transmission, at the present time, is the use of telephone lines for video conferencing. Two-way interactive video and audio communication is possible through fiber optic cables. *Fiber optic networks* have been developed in most states, connecting schools, higher education institutions, hospitals, governmental agencies, and other community organizations. These fiber optic networks offer very high quality, full-motion video conferencing at a far lower cost than current satellite technology. If participants have access to network sites, a fiber optic video conference is an exciting way to conduct a needs assessment exercise. Developing a network does require an extensive financial investment, however, to establish dedicated telephone lines between a limited number of fixed sites. Inter-network connections are possible, allowing for communication with additional sites separated by greater distances, but they require additional coordination and financial investment.

Another use of telephone lines for conferencing relies on *compressed video* technology. Unlike with fiber optic networks, compressed video is not limited to established fixed sites. Instead of using dedicated telephone lines, anyone with the appropriate equipment and technical expertise can use regular telephone lines to connect to a compressed video conference. Participants can dial another site directly or use a video bridge to connect several sites. The bridge simply manages all incoming and outgoing calls.

Establishing a compressed video system requires considerably less financial investment than creating a dedicated fiber optic network, but users typically incur long-distance toll charges for two to six telephone lines whenever the system is used. Recently, conducting a compressed video conference over the Internet has become possible, saving the long-distance telephone costs. Using telephone lines is still the preferred method at this time, however, because the connection is more stable than one established via the Internet.

Although compressed video is less costly and more agile than fiber optics, the quality is not as good. The major disadvantage is that at lower transmission rates, the video image can appear "jerky." Audio communication is also delayed slightly. Transmission of still images and graphics is usually of good quality. Users can choose the transmission rate they prefer, but all connecting sites must receive and transmit at the same rate. A higher transmission rate results in higher-quality video and audio communication, but the additional telephone lines needed mean higher long-distance charges. Compressed video conferencing has improved significantly in recent years, resulting in considerably less audio and video delay, and should develop further during this decade. It represents a promising approach to needs assessment, because participants potentially can use regular telephone lines or the Internet to connect anywhere in the world.

Even more promising is another form of video conferencing called *desktop conferencing*. Using the Internet, video images are transmitted and received through a regular personal computer monitor or through a small video monitor mounted on top of the computer monitor. Desktop video conferencing is a form of compressed video conferencing, albeit one typically carried out at the slowest transmission speed. Picture quality is at best fair, but it at least provides live two-way video interaction. Due to the widespread use of personal computers, desktop conferencing is potentially much more accessible for needs assessment exercises than compressed video systems or fiber optic networks. Improvements in compressed video technology in the years ahead should improve the quality of desktop conferencing as well.

Advantages

1. *More extensive interaction.* A video conference enables both verbal and nonverbal communication and provides opportunities to transmit graphics, videotapes, and other forms of multimedia.
2. *Typically a shorter process than a face-to-face meeting.* "Dial-up" long-distance charges for compressed video conferences, tightly scheduled transmission and reception facilities, and "technology fatigue" from using a more structured mode of communication all limit the length of a video conference.
3. *Attractive to busy people.* Even if travel to a special facility is necessary, the time and expense are usually less than those required for an extended face-to-face meeting.

Disadvantages

1. *Less accessible.* People can participate in a conference call in the office, at home, or at other locations, but a video conference often requires a specially equipped facility. Many people currently do not have access to these facilities.
2. *Significantly more expensive.* Developing a fiber optic network requires a major capital investment. Once established, long-distance communication is available at no cost to network members, but the network may charge user fees to recover overhead costs. Compressed video equipment is less costly, but the long-distance charges for

multiple telephone lines add up. Participants typically need technical support when using video conferencing equipment, which also adds to the cost.

3. *Requires more advance planning.* A video conference usually requires reserving a specially equipped room and scheduling time on a network or securing the use of a video bridge.

4. *More limited nonverbal communication than in a face-to-face meeting.* Picture quality for compressed video conferencing varies considerably, depending on the transmission speed. The video and audio delay makes facial expressions more difficult to decipher. Fiber optic video conferences have better picture quality, but subtle forms of nonverbal communication are less obvious.

5. *Occasional awkward verbal communication with compressed video and desktop conferencing.* Participants can see a speaker at another location but experience a slight delay hearing what is said. When viewing someone responding to a question, they may wonder at first if the respondent heard the question. Delayed audio communication also affects humor. Just when a speaker begins to conclude that a joke apparently fell flat, reassuring laughter saves embarrassment.

Despite the apparent disadvantages of video conferencing, take heart. The advantage of two-way video communication is very significant for communication at a distance. The improvements in this technology that will occur in the years ahead and its expansion into ever more schools, hospitals, governmental agencies, businesses, and nonprofit organizations should result in its widespread use for needs assessment activities.

Preparing for the Assessment

As with any needs and capacity assessment strategy, several general steps are necessary to prepare for the assessment. For example, you need to select the participants and develop the issues on which to focus. Additional specific steps are necessary to prepare for audio, computer, and video conferencing.

1. *Schedule the conference for the convenience of most participants.* If you are using a dedicated audio or video network, or even an audio or video bridge, you must consider the time available on those systems. Dialing each participant directly offers the most flexible scheduling.

A computer conference requires arranging for computer time and specifying the time frame during which people must respond to your information. Stivers, Bently, and Meccouri (1995) list some of the more frequently used public health-related discussion lists and online discussion groups available.

2. *Select one or two major questions to consider during the conference.* Because several people will participate, you cannot ask as many questions as during a telephone survey. You will need to allow time for everyone to respond to your questions and time for the participants to respond to one another, if desired. The people who participate in these conferences are often busy, so you want to use the time you have to best advantage.

3. *Prepare graphics, videotapes, and other multimedia materials as appropriate.* These enhancements add variety and quality to a video conference and counter the tendency to rely on "talking heads."

4. *Send the participants information in advance of the conference.* Remind them when the conference will take place, who it includes, and what you hope to accomplish. If possible, list the questions you plan to ask, so that they can think about how to respond.

5. *Schedule training and technical support as needed.* Participants in a video conference need instructions, demonstrations, and practice in using the equipment, preferably before the conference actually begins. Otherwise, valuable time will be wasted. In the worst case, untrained and inexperienced participants could sabotage the entire video conference. If possible, arrange for technical support personnel to be present or close by during the conference to handle any technical problems that arise.

Conducting the Assessment

1. *Use the first few minutes for warm up.* Start the conference on time, but do not plunge into the first question right away. Instead, introduce yourself and restate the purpose of the conference. Conduct a roll call to ensure that everyone who is to be involved is on the line. This roll call also gives each person the opportunity to become comfortable with the equipment and to make sure it is operating satisfactorily.

2. *Ask your questions in a structured fashion.* One option is to ask a question and then proceed to call on each person by name for a response. A structured approach is important for audio conferencing because you cannot observe facial clues to determine who is ready to respond. Interjecting comments during an audio conference is also more difficult than during a face-to-face meeting. Less spontaneous people may have trouble making their comments if they are not asked directly. By comparison, the discussion will likely flow more easily during a video conference.

After everyone has had an opportunity to respond, pause and ask whether anyone has any other comments to add before moving to the next question. If possible, try to summarize what the group has said before discussing the next question.

Less structure is necessary for a small group, especially if the members are relatively comfortable with one another. It is possible to throw the question out to the group and let the participants respond. Before moving to another question, though, be sure to ask those who have not responded if they have any comments.

3. *Record the information.* If at all possible, try to have someone other than the conference moderator present during an audio conference to take extensive notes. That leaves the moderator free to concentrate on conducting the conference. Tape recording is another possibility for an audio or video conference when the issues are not sensitive, provided that the group is clearly informed of its use. Recording information is less of a challenge for computer conferencing, as the written dialogue is easily stored or printed.

Using the Results

As soon after the conference as possible, summarize the information gathered. Because the conference has been conducted in a structured manner, this summary should be easy to organize. If possible, send the summary to the participants. Ask them to review it for accuracy and send you any corrections needed. Then share the information with your planning committee.

Undoubtedly, the explosion in technology we are experiencing at the present time is creating exciting possibilities for examining health-related needs. Additional possibilities are on the horizon. Of some concern, however, is whether these advances will primarily benefit more affluent populations at the expense of less affluent individuals. Such a development would require judicious use of technology to assess needs of certain populations, so as to avoid bias in the results.

Reviewing an Example

A computer-mediated communication (CMC) process used at Central Queensland University, Australia, for the discussion of a case study with off-campus postgraduate students (professionals involved in continuing education) is described by Gregor and Cuskelly (1994). Although it was a course-related experience, the authors describe the value of the e-mail exchanges that resulted. The process is characterized as informal and not dominated by stronger personalities due to the technology used for the communications. The authors note that having participants communicate their perspectives on a focused issue was well suited for the bulletin board approach, and that "short notices and contributions may be better assimilated than lengthier contributions" (p. 178).

The participants had from six months to more than two years of computer experience, with the majority citing the greater level of experience. The authors believe, however, that the less experienced users were not inhibited from using the computer technology. Additionally, based on the results of a follow-up questionnaire, the majority of the participants believed that the bulletin board process facilitated more "discussion" than usual, and there was an openness toward using the format in other ways.

Online Resources

Visit http://healtheducation.jbpub.com/gilmore for links to these Web sites.

Agency for Health Care Research and Quality
A Web-assisted audio conference on surge capacity assessments and regionalization issues.

National Information Center on Health Services Research and Health Care Technology
Outlines the ten basic steps to health care research assessments.

UNC School of Public Health
Information on video conferencing.

VA Great Lakes
Information on video conferencing, telemedicine, and audiovisual equipment.

National Network for Child Care, Videoconference
An example of a videoconference evaluation.

References

Dutta, P., Jena, T., and Panda, S. (1996). A Plea for Health Manpower Training Through Distance Education. *Medical Education Online*, 1, 8 (http://www.Med-Ed-Online.org).

Gregor, S., and Cuskelly, E. (1994). Computer Mediated Communication in Distance Education. *Journal of Computer Assisted Learning*, 10, 168–181.

Stivers, C., Bently, M., and Meccouri, L. (1995). Internet: The Contemporary Health Educator's Most Versatile Tool. *Journal of Health Education*, 26, 196–199.

Large-Scale Community Assessment Strategies

Introduction

Over the last decade, several needs and capacity assessment procedures have emerged that are applied to communities and regions as part of a larger health planning framework. These large-scale community assessment strategies typically are highly planned, resource-intensive, and long-term in nature. A number of those that we will describe here are based on collaborative efforts involving both the public and the private sectors. They strive for a variety of approaches to assessment that will yield insights into diverse populations within a specified geographic area.

Reviewing the Strategies

The following community needs and capacity assessment strategies are current examples of large-scale approaches. The assessment components are part of a larger planning framework. They have been developed through the collaborative efforts of several agencies and organizations, and have been implemented in community settings for a number of years. The major *advantages* of these approaches are that they (1) provide a comprehensive review of the needs and strengths of the population, (2) tie into a planning framework that includes the development and implementation of action plans, and (3) encourage partnerships and collaborative efforts among organizations and community members. The major *disadvantages* are that they (1) are very time-intensive, (2) are highly resource-intensive, and (3) require continual monitoring and maintenance to keep the process moving and individuals motivated to participate in the various committee procedures. A few key large-scale frameworks and their salient characteristics are described below.

Assessment Protocol for Excellence in Public Health (APEX-PH)

With the financial support of the National Association of County Health Officials and the Centers for Disease Control and Prevention, six professional and official organizations joined together to develop an assessment process intended for use by local health departments entitled the Assessment Protocol for Excellence in Public Health (**APEX-PH**) (CDC, 2003; National Association of County Health Officials, 1991). This approach was developed in a response to several national reports that emphasized the need for a focus on prevention and health promotion (e.g., *Healthy People 2010*) as well as the important role played by local health departments in conducting needs assessments, policy development, and assurance activities (Institute of Medicine, 2003).

The process consists of three parts. In the first phase, an organizational capacity assessment addresses how an agency can review and improve its performance. An eight-step process is recommended that seeks to analyze an organization's strengths and weaknesses and then to rank order problems according to three criteria: magnitude of the problem, seriousness of the consequences of the problem, and feasibility of correcting the problem. Afterward, a plan can be developed to strengthen the organization's status. Worksheets are provided to assist in the organizational assessment.

The second phase involves the community assessment process, in which the organization works with the community, particularly through a community health committee, to identify, prioritize, and analyze community health problems. Worksheets are provided to assist in identifying health problems through a review of secondary information—particularly demographic, morbidity, and mortality data. In addition, the community health committee is encouraged to serve as a sounding board by reacting to the proposed community health problems suggested by the organization's staff. The selection of a prioritization process in which community health problems are ranked is open to the discretion of the organization's staff and the committee. The nominal group process with its systematic ranking is one recommended approach.

Also included in the second phase is an analysis component, which delves into why a particular health problem exists by reviewing its risk factors (scientifically established determinants that relate directly to the level of a health problem—for example, low birth weight as an influence on infant mortality), direct contributing factors (scientifically established determinants that directly affect the level of a risk factor—for example, teen pregnancy as an influence on low birth weight), and indirect contributing factors (community-specific determinants that directly affect the level of direct contributing factors—for example, low self-esteem as an influence on teen pregnancy). Based on this information as well as a review of actual and potential resources, the committee can develop a specific community health plan for implementation.

The third phase addresses activities that will support the implementation of the plan of action. These include policy development procedures, assurances of continuing support for the community health committee, ongoing data surveillance, public health service provision, monitoring of progress, and formal evaluation of the effectiveness in meeting the stated goals and objectives in the plan.

Planned Approach to Community Health (PATCH)

The origins of the Planned Approach to Community Health (PATCH) date back to the early 1980s, when the then-titled Center for Health Promotion and Education in the Centers for Disease Control and Prevention attempted to guide the proposal development and support efforts of the Health Education–Risk Reduction (HERR) categorical grants program (CDC, 2002). Even as this federal categorical grant process evolved into a more state-managed prevention block grant approach with the addition of seven other categorical grant programs, the overriding principle remained encouraging the development of an organized, planned approach to community-based interventions by local, state, and federal health organizations (Kreuter, 1992). The two original goals that continue to direct the PATCH efforts today are (1) to "create a practical mechanism through which effective community health education action could be targeted to address local level health priorities," and (2) to "offer a practical, skill-based program of technical assistance wherein health education leaders in state health agencies would work with their local health counterparts to establish community health education programs" (Kreuter, 1992, p. 136).

The PATCH approach incorporates a community intervention strategy within the context of the PRECEDE model described in Chapter 2. Indeed, it was the emerging PATCH process that "inspired the PROCEED expansion of the model to encompass policy, regulatory, and organizational issues of program implementation" (Green and Kreuter, 1992, p. 143). With national leadership from the Centers for Disease Control and Prevention, PATCH works with national partners from voluntary agencies, Cooperative Extension, and the National Education Association. More than 42 states, the District of Columbia, the Virgin Islands, and international sites such as Queensland, Australia (CDC, 2002; Swannell, Steele, Harvey, et al., 1992), participate in the PATCH network, including both civilian and military populations. The framework for activity involves vertical (national to local level) and horizontal (across the various partnership agencies and organizations) communications and support (see **Figure 1**).

The driving force behind the approach is the encouragement of local ownership. Particularly during the needs assessment phase, which encompasses an average of one year of data collection and analysis, a sense of empowerment emerges as involved individuals and groups come to realize that they are a part of the decision-making process. **Figure 2** depicts the usual steps in the PATCH process that precede the determination of health promotion needs and community diagnosis methods, followed up with the identification of

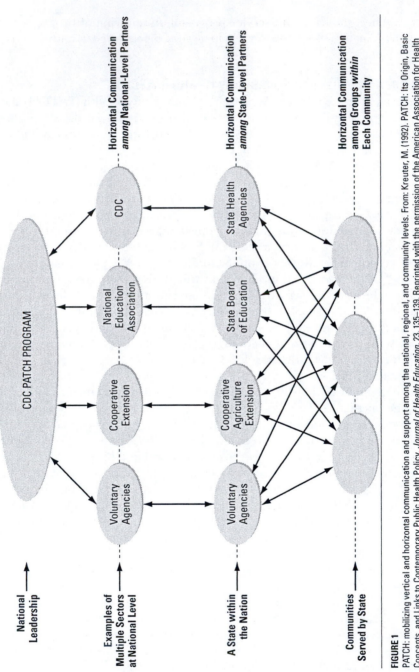

National
Leadership →

Examples of
Multiple Sectors →
at National Level

A State within →
the Nation

Communities →
Served by State

CDC PATCH PROGRAM

Voluntary Agencies

Cooperative Extension

National Education Association

CDC

Horizontal Communication *among* National-Level Partners

Voluntary Agencies

Cooperative Agriculture Extension

State Board of Education

State Health Agencies

Horizontal Communication *among* State-Level Partners

Horizontal Communication among Groups *within* Each Community

FIGURE 1
PATCH: mobilizing vertical and horizontal communication and support among the national, regional, and community levels. From: Kreuter, M. (1992). PATCH: Its Origin, Basic Concepts, and Links to Contemporary Public Health Policy. *Journal of Health Education, 23,* 135–139. Reprinted with the permission of the American Association for Health Education.

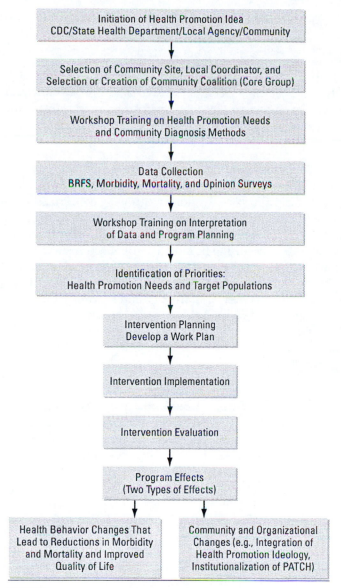

FIGURE 2
The presumptive PATCH model. From: Steckler, A., Orville, K., Eng, E., and Dawson, L. (1992). Summary of a Formative Evaluation of PATCH. *Journal of Health Education*, 23, 174–178. Reprinted with the permission of the American Association for Health Education.

priorities for work plan development. Five elements in PATCH are considered critical:

1. Community members participate in the process.
2. Data guide the development of programs.
3. Participants develop a comprehensive health promotion strategy.
4. Evaluation emphasizes feedback and program improvement.
5. The community capacity for health promotion is increased (CDC, 2002).

This approach is exemplified by the effort undertaken by the National Coalition of Hispanic Health and Human Service Organizations, which selected the PATCH approach to address a growing concern about the leading causes of death among Hispanics in El Paso, Texas (Ugarte, Duarte, and Wilson, 1992). The approach taken was considered unique because the assessment strategies needed to be modified to reflect the bilingual, bicultural, and unique health needs of that population and resulted in the development of the Hispanic Health Needs Assessment (HHNA) process. It incorporated a community profile, review of morbidity and mortality rates, a behavioral risk factor survey, and community opinion surveys for local leaders and residents. It was felt that the comprehensive assessment approach was an important first step in being able to initiate health promotion programs in Hispanic communities.

Mobilizing for Action through Planning and Partnerships (MAPP)

An emerging large-scale process with key needs and capacity assessment phases is the community-wide strategic planning tool known as Mobilizing for Action through Planning and Partnerships (MAPP); it is offered through the National Association of County and City Health Officials in cooperation with the Centers for Disease Control and Prevention (www.naccho.org/tools.cfm). The process begins with communities bringing various partners together for organizational and shared visioning purposes. These steps are followed by the community's involvement in four key needs and capacity assessments:

- Community themes and strengths, which identifies community assets, interests, and perceptions about quality of life;
- Local public health system assessment, which measures the capacity and performance of the local public health system along with other community organizations;
- Community health status assessment, which assesses health status, quality of life, and risk factor data; and
- Forces of change assessment, which identifies forces affecting the community or the local public health system (www.naccho.org/tools.cfm).

Following the various assessment phases, an illustrated community roadmap is developed so that all stakeholders can envision a healthier community as a destination: "moving along a road that leads to a healthier community" (NACCHO, 2003, p. 1). Currently, nine demonstration sites throughout the United States are preparing for and implementing the MAPP process so that review and revision can take place.

COMPASS Community Assessment

United Way of America has developed a community-based needs and capacity assessment process that enables representatives from community agencies to become engaged in comprehensive planning, implementation, and evaluation procedures. The process, called **Community COMPASS**, is presently in its second iteration (version 2.0). Six communities in the United States (e.g., La Crosse, Wisconsin) used the earlier version of the needs and asset assessment process, and their feedback led to the revisions and updates in the subsequent version. This approach draws upon key community resource materials developed earlier by United Way (United Way of America, 1996, 1997). Some local public health agencies have found it of value to use the collaborative COMPASS approach as their community-wide needs and asset assessment process while developing their community health strategic plans (personal communication, Douglas Mormann, La Crosse County Health Department, 2003).

Healthworks

Developed by the Erie County (Pennsylvania) Department of Health for the assessment of citizens' health promotion needs and interests in small community settings ranging from 5,000 to 20,000 in population size, **Healthworks** particularly focuses on weight control, nutrition, exercise, smoking cessation, and seat-belt use. The assessment approach incorporates a Health Risk Appraisal, a 17-item Health Knowledge and Opinion survey instrument, and the health screening measures of height, weight, blood pressure, and cholesterol level. The developers of the format acknowledge that the process is designed to assess major health risks without attempting a comprehensive analysis of the community health needs (Erie County Department of Health, 1992).

Ten steps in the process are described, starting with the selection of a coordinator and support staff. This step is followed by developing a draft implementation plan, selecting a target community, identifying the target audience, marshalling resources, selecting survey instruments and screening methods, gaining support from community leaders, forming a steering committee, soliciting the donation of incentive prizes, and scheduling of town meetings and feedback sessions so that citizens have multiple opportunities to learn about the results and planned action measures. This approach allows for a good deal of flexibility in selecting alternative resources and assessment formats.

Preparing for the Assessment

All of the large-scale community assessment formats require carefully established timelines with several months of lead time built in. Additionally, if grant-related funding will be sought, one must plan one to two years in advance of the assessment implementation phase to prepare the appropriate proposals.

While the timelines certainly will vary depending on the size of the population base, the degree of difficulty in accessing and working with partners and the target audience, and the availability of resources, the approach offered by Healthworks does offer a helpful preliminary planning framework:

Six to nine months before kick-off:

1. Select a coordinator and support staff.
2. Develop a draft implementation plan.
3. Select a target community.
4. Define your target audience.
5. Marshall your resources.

Three to six months before kick-off:

6. Select your survey instruments and screening methods.
7. Gain support from community leaders.
8. Form a steering committee.
9. Solicit donations of incentive prizes.
10. Schedule town meetings and feedback sessions (p. 5).

It is important to add to this list that the early review of secondary data regarding, at a minimum, the demographics, morbidity, and mortality information for a community will yield valuable insights. The worksheets provided for the APEX-PH process can facilitate this phase in terms of its logical data collection format and its ability to provide for data reporting to committee members.

Those wishing to learn more about the PATCH approach, given its extensive national, state, and local partnership configuration, can contact the Division of Chronic Disease Control and Community Intervention at the National Center for Chronic Disease Prevention and Health Promotion, Centers for Disease Control and Prevention, located in Atlanta, Georgia.

Conducting the Assessment

In addition to having an established timeline with aligned responsibilities, it will be essential to have mutually agreed-upon means of communication with all partners during the assessment implementation phase. Written timeline/responsibility information, secondary data summaries, meeting summaries, and the sharing and discussion of preliminary primary data findings will need to be built into the assessment process. This effort will ensure that all of the partners are kept as up-to-date as possible while the assessment progresses, and will enable revisions in the process to occur as needed. Data updates should be scheduled as routinely as the steering committee deems appropriate.

Due to the multiple assessment procedures that usually are incorporated into large-scale community-based approaches, it is recommended that assessment purpose statements be established to guide the methods selected. One example would be "to characterize the living standards of this population," which could be addressed through a review of that population's demographic data.

Using the Results

The large-scale community assessment formats occur within the context of a larger planning framework. For that reason, the collected needs information can be fed directly into the action planning phase of the respective framework. Typically, this entails the prioritization of the assessed needs using established criteria (see Chapter 2), leading to the development of overarching goals and action-related objectives for health enhancement. Note that while the data sources are valuable in gaining insights into the needs of the population, the discussion that ensues from steering, planning, and/or advisory committees reviewing such information represents a rich resource of ideas, concerns, and issues that should not be taken lightly. These inputs can be particularly welcome contributions as one attempts to derive trends and patterns from the multiple data sources. Over time, you should learn to trust the instincts and insights of a longstanding, representative committee that is being properly facilitated.

Reviewing an Example

A rural health promotion project was established in Vernon County, Wisconsin, to demonstrate that health care providers could work in partnership with community organizations to identify health needs and then mutually address those needs (Gilmore, Traastad, and Johnson, 2003; Favor, Robinson, and Gilmore, 1994). Representatives from these organizations were members of the Community Health Intervention Partnership (CHIPs) Council, which served as the oversight and planning body. It was suggested that seven clustered, but not mutually exclusive, target groups be addressed in the effort: Amish, youth, elderly, farming families, unemployed, socioeconomically disadvantaged, and general public.

The planning framework deemed most appropriate for the county-wide effort was the APEX-PH approach, with certain modifications in the organizational assessment phase. Because all of the organizations represented on the CHIPs Council had interacted with one another previously, a general sense of trust was already engendered, as was an understanding of available resources. Following the collection and review of public and private sources of secondary data, a survey was developed, pilot tested, and implemented in the county. The survey assessed general well-being, risk factor and protective factor involvement, social networking opportunities, environmental factors, and personal, family, and community health promotional issues within a sample population ranging in age from 13 to 103 years. Additional insights into the top-priority health issues were revealed through a nominal group meeting of selected citizens from throughout the county who represented the seven target populations. Based on a continuing review of these primary and secondary data sources, the CHIPs Council was able to identify three top-priority areas for immediate attention to be addressed through the development and implementation of action plans, as coordinated by respective subcommittees: (1) enhancement of primary prevention and health promotion activities, (2) strengthening of the family unit, and (3) improvement of access to services and information.

The overall effort was deemed a success due to the continuing nature of the CHIPs Council as the three-year foundation funding concluded, the enduring partnerships that were established across the county, the sense of trust and resource sharing that prevailed, and the successful accomplishment of many of the outcomes specified in the action plans. During the 1999–2002 period, the needs and capacity assessment process was repeated using a revised survey format, followed by action plan development for the county during 2003.

Online Resources

Visit http://healtheducation.jbpub.com/gilmore for links to these Web sites.

Assessment Protocol for Excellence in Public Health (APEX)
Overview of APEX-PH process with contact information.

Study Circles Research Center
Documentation and assessment of the community-wide study circles and best practices links.

Higher Education Center for Alcohol and Other Drug Prevention
Statewide initiative assessment, strategic planning, and evaluation.

Centers for Disease Control and Prevention
CDC Assessment Protocol for Excellence in Public Health (APEX) publication and links.

APEX
A PowerPoint presentation on APEX presented by NACCHO and the CDC in alignment with the three core public health functions.

PATCH
CDC PATCH document presented and described, to include a guide for the local coordinator.

References

Centers for Disease Control and Prevention (CDC), Division of Public Health Surveillance and Informatics. (2003). *Assessment Protocol for Excellence in Public Health (APEX-PH)*. Atlanta, GA. http://wonder.cdc.gov/wonder/prevguid/p0000089/p0000089.asp.

Centers for Disease Control and Prevention (CDC), National Center for Chronic Disease Prevention and Health Promotion. (2002). *PATCH: A Guide for the Local Coordinator*. Atlanta, GA. http://www.cdc.gov/nccdphp/patch/.

Erie County Department of Health. (1992). *Healthworks: Guide for Conducting a Community-Based Health Risk Appraisal Program*. Erie, PA.

Favor, S., Robinson, J., and Gilmore, G. (1994). *Report of the Vernon County Community Health Intervention Project*. Westby, WI: Coulee CAP.

Gilmore, G., Traastad, K., and Johnson, E. (2003). *Vernon County, Wisconsin, Health Needs Assessment Report: 1999–2002*. University of Wisconsin–Extension.

Green, L., and Kreuter, M. (1992). CDC's Planned Approach to Community Health as an Application of PRECEDE and an Inspiration for PROCEED. *Journal of Health Education*, 23, 140–144.

Institute of Medicine. (2003). *The Future of the Public's Health in the 21st Century*. Washington, DC: National Academies Press.

Kreuter, M. (1992). PATCH: Its Origins, Basic Concepts, and Links to Contemporary Public Health Policy. *Journal of Health Education*, 23, 135–139.

National Association of County and City Health Officials. (1991). *Assessment Protocol for Excellence in Public Health*. Washington, DC.

Swannell, R., Steele, J., Harvey, P., Bruggemann, J., Town, S., Emery, E., and Schmid, T. (1992). PATCH in Australia: Elements of a Successful Implementation. *Journal of Health Education*, 23, 171–173.

Ugarte, C., Duarte, P., and Wilson, K. (1992). PATCH as a Model for Development of an Hispanic Health Needs Assessment: The El Paso Experience. *Journal of Health Education*, 23, 153–156.

United Way of America. (1997). *ACCESS97: User's Guide*. Alexandria, VA.

United Way of America. (1996). *Measuring Program Outcomes: A Practical Approach*. Alexandria, VA.

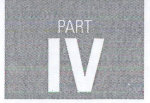

Self-Directed Assessments

Self-directed assessments are personal review procedures. A majority of these approaches address primary prevention issues, such as the assessment of risk factors and protective factors in one's lifestyle pattern, and the secondary prevention process of the early detection of disease symptoms. Some of these strategies combine the two aspects of prevention so that risk factors and symptoms can be detected and addressed. Still others expand into an assessment of positive (protective) factors in one's lifestyle, thereby becoming more wellness oriented (e.g., assessing positive exercise, diet, and relaxation patterns). Although some of the assessment procedures, such as breast self-examination, require initial instruction, others do not (taking a self-scored General Health Status Inventory, for example). Some of the assessment inventories are self-scored, whereas others are computer analyzed. In Chapters 11 and 12, we will review a variety of approaches for health and wellness assessment.

Self-Directed Assessment Inventories

Introduction

Individual concern for heightened levels of wellness and willingness to take personal responsibility for certain lifestyle changes have been the recent focus on health promotion in our society. Although the degree of individual commitment and follow-through varies greatly, it is clear that a rather potent health consciousness has arisen in our society.

Several key efforts have been designed to kindle national concern about health and overall well-being. Notable among these is *Healthy People 2010* (2000), which provides national objectives for health promotion and disease prevention. It clarifies the risks to good health, including those lifestyle aspects over which an individual has a good deal of control—for example, smoking, alcohol misuse and abuse, poor diet, lack of regular exercise, and stress. While the initiative largely focuses on risk factors and disease and injury outcome reduction, guided by a "determinants of health" approach, the framework also targets certain protective factors, such as eating a balanced diet, engaging in physical activity, and establishing healthy schools and worksites. The report calls for more attention to be paid to multiple levels of responsibility involving individuals, families, health professionals, health institutions, schools, business and labor, communities, and government. Particular attention is centered on the individual's role in making day-to-day decisions. Importantly, the public needs to be reminded about the value of health screenings as a complement to primary prevention strategies (i.e., preventive efforts taken before a particular disease develops). Organizations like the American Cancer Society continue to explore viable options to convey essential screening messages to the public, through information systems and program activity (personal communication, Cynthia Currence, National Vice President for Strategic Corporate Marketing Alliances, American Cancer Society, October 28, 2003).

This chapter examines health promotion assessment inventories that can be used with individuals, to be potentially followed up with intervention, planned change, or strategies and their reinforcement (Powers and Dodd, 2003;

Squire, Gilmore, Duquette, and Riley, 2001; Gilmore, Dosch, and Hood, 1985; Gilmore, 1979). Some of the available formats provide a brief assessment of several health promotional dimensions, known as general health status inventories (GHSIs). The basic intent of these formats is to quickly sensitize an individual to risk factor considerations, typically through self-scoring and interpretation. More in-depth risk factor assessments are available through health risk appraisals (HRAs), which are usually longer and scored by computer. Both formats tend to concentrate almost exclusively on risk factors, or disease/death/disability inducers. In a third type of format, provided by wellness inventories (WIs), risk factors and protective factors, or health-related inducers, are assessed (Squire, Gilmore, Duquette, and Riley, 2001; Gilmore, Dosch, and Hood, 1985).

The groundings for these types of assessments are described in a brief historical sketch by Hall and Zwemer (1979). They cite the landmark efforts by Dr. Lewis Robbins, who, while serving as Chief of the U.S. Public Health Service Cancer Control Program, fostered the development of a preventive approach that would identify and appraise disease precursors, eventually leading to risk reduction efforts. In 1959, 25 health risk appraisals were completed at the Department of Preventive Medicine at Temple University School of Medicine, incorporating the probability tables (chances of dying) which had been developed by Harvey Geller, then a statistician with the Cancer Control Program. By 1962, the term "prospective medicine" had been coined.

These events eventually led to a series of key events:

- The publication of *How to Practice Prospective Medicine* in 1970 by Robbins and Hall
- Early use of prospective medicine in Canada, starting in 1971
- The incorporation of the Society of Prospective Medicine in 1974
- A collaborative agreement between the U.S. Centers for Disease Control (CDC) and Health and Welfare Canada for further health risk appraisal research and development in 1978
- The first CDC Health Risk Appraisal Users Conference to stimulate the use of the process and to share information in 1983
- The introduction of a reformulated version of the adult HRA in 1987

Reviewing and Selecting a Strategy

General Health Status Inventories

One simple process for health promotional assessment involves self-scored general health appraisals. These usually brief, self-reported, hand-scored inventories address a few health promotion categories, such as cigarette smoking, alcohol and drug use, diet and fitness, stress management, and safety. Using very few questions or statements in each category, this process attempts to develop preliminary sensitization to selected risk factors and protective factors. It is helpful in initially directing the attention of an individual or group toward prevention and health promotion issues, to be followed with an educational message and possibly certain health promotional activities. If the individual or group is to be involved in additional sessions, more advanced assessment procedures, such as those described later in this chapter, could be employed.

Examples of GHSIs include *Healthstyle*, originally developed by the U.S. Department of Health and Human Services (see Appendix A); the "Living Smart Quiz" by the American Cancer Society, which briefly assesses one's dietary and activity patterns; and a host of lifestyle assessments for various audiences (e.g., see Powers and Dodd, 2003).

Computer-Analyzed Health Risk Appraisals

A more in-depth analysis of health risks is provided by computer-analyzed health risk appraisals. This appraisal format typically relies on participant self-reported information related to demographics; use of tobacco, alcohol, and other drugs; use of seat belts; involvement in physical activity; use of disease screening activities (for example, a Pap smear); hazardous practices (such as hitchhiking); and a brief health history.

The original health risk appraisals, offered through the CDC, were based on an actuarial model incorporating national mortality statistics related to age, gender, and race (white or nonwhite). The printout from this format provided individualized information about one's chances of dying within the next ten years from each of 12 ranked causes of death per 100,000 population. A summary of these data yielded an appraised health age (an estimate of how healthy one is in comparison to others of the same race, age, and gender) and an achievable age (an estimate of how healthy one could be if recommended lifestyle changes are made). For example, if a 45-year-old Caucasian man is informed that his appraised health age is 49 years, the risk factors in his lifestyle align him with the death statistics of Caucasian men aged four years older. If he was willing to alter some of those risk factors, it could result in an achieved health age of 45 years. The printout provides information about recommended lifestyle changes based on the risk factors, as well as an expanded review of each possible cause of death and related risk categories.

While early versions of the HRA used the paper-and-pencil method for recording an individual's health risk information, electronic technology has advanced the process into the twenty-first century. Gorsky (2003) has addressed the changes that have taken place over time in going from a paper-based HRA to Internet and palm-based formats (see Appendix B). His review concludes that each format can have a place, depending on the audiences and settings to be accessed. Health promotion assessment instruments and HRAs are described in Appendix D.

Wellness Inventories

Another grouping of health assessments includes wellness inventories. These formats are typically self-reported, computer-scored inventories that address a broad spectrum of health-related factors and their effects on morbidity, mortality, and health enhancement. Here the health-related factors can be either risk factors (leading to negative impacts in a person's life), or protective factors (leading to positive impacts). A number of the available formats are described by Beery et al. (1986). As with HRAs, these types of assessments need to be reviewed for reliability (consistency) and validity (accuracy).

One example of a wellness inventory is the La Crosse Wellness Inventory (LWI), which is part of the La Crosse Wellness Project (see Appendix C). The inventory was developed as a wellness assessment format to be included in the overall process of assessment, intervention, and reinforcement. Initiated through the efforts of a community planning committee in 1976, the LWI—along with its follow-up, intervention, and reinforcement procedures—has been researched in university and community settings. Its primary content validity was established through a national jury process. Its overall reliability (internal consistency) was calculated at 0.87 (Gilmore, et al., 1983; Gilmore, Dosch, and Hood, 1985). Additional types of WIs and information for ordering them are listed in Appendix E.

The development of WIs usually follows a four-step process: (1) formulating questions based on literature reviews, (2) refining the questions, (3) validating the questions through comparisons with standards, and (4) calculating reliability coefficients. Richardson (1986) notes that this process is more appropriate when epidemiologic data are not available for diverse lifestyle factors such as frustration, adaptive stress, and depression. With WIs, the goal is to assess areas of health-related strengths and weaknesses. It is not to determine the length of one's life based on health practices.

Preparing for the Assessment

There are a few major considerations when preparing to use self-directed assessment inventories. First, these inventories are not self-reliant. They can be but one part of a total program experience, one type of assessment. Other program aspects, such as intervention and reinforcement, will need attention as well (McKenzie and Smeltzer, 1997; Hyer and Melby, 1985).

Second, individualized explanation, interpretation, and behavioral counseling regarding the inventory results are beneficial. It is not recommended to involve participants in GHSIs without follow-up discussion or to send HRA and WI results through the mail. Depending on the program's focus, time should be allocated for a clarification of the meaning of the results, particularly for the HRA and WI, including discussions about individualized steps or strategies for health-related changes.

Third, multiple program sessions appear to enhance the impact on participants, in contrast to singular events (Gilmore, Dosch, and Hood, 1985; Hyer and Melby, 1985). Repeated sessions allow time not only for the necessary inventory analyses, but also for more in-depth individualized discussion regarding the meaning of the results and possible next steps.

Fourth, these assessment inventories are not solely aligned with one professional group. Although they have their groundings in epidemiological research and physician-to-patient counseling, they have been routinely incorporated into programming by health departments, business and industry (Abby, 1986), insurance companies, voluntary agencies, and other private agencies (Hyer and Melby, 1985).

Fifth, HRAs can be used to create community risk assessments (as distinguished from individualized appraisal) through the calculation of the population, attributable risk proportion (PARP), as presented in Appendix G. This approach allows for the review of the impact on a population of risk factor combinations over time.

Finally, HRAs are targeted primarily for mainstream, employed, literate adults, even though other target groups serve as major reservoirs of preventable risks (Moriarty, 1986; Rowley, et al., 1986). As a consequence, caution should be exercised in considering the use of these assessments with underrepresented populations. The assessments can be incorporated quite easily into employee health promotion programs. One example would be with the American Cancer Society's "Active for Life" Program, which is a 10-week program encouraging people to be more active on a regular basis (ACS, 2002). Individual assessments can be used to enable participants to set their own goals based on how currently active they are in relation to how active they want to be in the future. The assessments can be repeated at various intervals to record one's progress.

Various characteristics of the three inventory formats are detailed in **Table 1**. Usually, the HRA and WI formats will be more in-depth than the GHSI. Keep

TABLE 1
Characteristics of Three Assessment Inventory Formats

	GHSI	HRA	WI
Assessment purpose	General health awareness	Risk of dying in next ten years	Health strengths and weaknesses
Type of reinforcement	Negative	Negative	Negative and positive
Scoring process	Self-scored	Computer-scored and self-scored	Computer-scored and self-scored
Administration process	One-time basis	Repeatable	Repeatable

in mind that the basic purpose of the GHSI is to catch the risk factors over which individuals have some control, as well as those unchangeable risk factors (e.g., heredity) that could encourage modified behaviors. The usual GHSI and HRA inventory formats focus on a negative reinforcement approach of avoiding hazards. The WI formats basically focus on positive and negative reinforcers so that undesirable behaviors can be reduced and desirable behaviors can be enhanced (Powers and Dodd, 2003; Gilmore, Dosch, and Hood, 1985; Hyer and Melby, 1985; Richardson, 1986).

Considerations for the implementation of the three inventory formats are cited in **Table 2**. One very important step prior to administering the HRA and WI formats is to make certain that enough advisors are trained for the explanation, interpretation, and counseling sessions. Typically, each advisor can work with as many as ten participants.

Plan and conduct an advisor training session that includes the following steps:

1. Advisors-to-be should take the inventory prior to your training session so that the printouts will be available on the date of the training.
2. During the training session, include participant and trainer introductions as well as a review of the training agenda (usually two trainers can work with up to 15 advisors-to-be).
3. Present a brief history of the inventory format (15 minutes).
4. Return and discuss the inventory results just as if the advisors-to-be were program participants, during the next 45 minutes to one hour.

TABLE 2
Implementation Considerations for Three Assessment Inventory Formats

	GHSI	HRA	WI
Preliminary steps	Identify target audience Secure site	Identify target audience Train advisors Secure site	Identify target audience Train advisors Secure site
Materials	Inventory Writing implements	Inventory Answer sheets Writing implements Computer	Inventory Answer sheets Writing implements Computer
Administration time	10 minutes	20–35 minutes	20–45 minutes
Interpretation time	15 minutes	30 minutes–1 hour	30 minutes–2 hours

5. Encourage questions for 15 to 30 minutes.
6. Discuss the process you would like the advisors to follow with the program participants during the next hour.
7. If there is enough time, demonstrate the computer program that was used to analyze the inventory responses and produce a printout.

Conducting the Assessment

After making the various logistical arrangements for the program, you will need to have the program participants take the HRA or WI in advance of the program date if it is a singular event (the GHSI can be taken on site) or at the first session of a multiple-session program. In contacting program participants in advance, send a letter with the inventory and answer sheet attachments that communicates the following message: This assessment is a very special feature of the program that will take approximately 25 minutes to complete; the results will be presented at the first program session and will be confidential; the assessment is a process for understanding the impact of one's health habits, and not a diagnostic process; from this a personal health promotion strategy can be developed; the inventory should be completed as accurately as possible because more complete responses will yield a clearer picture of the impact of one's health habits; and the answer sheet and the inventory should be returned by a specific date in an enclosed self-addressed, stamped envelope.

Many of these same ideas can be presented at the first session of a multiple-session program. It is particularly important to emphasize that the purpose of the assessment is to understand the impact of one's health habits, that accuracy of responses is important, and that the results are confidential. Participants can be informed that a follow-up session has been planned so their results can be returned, general principles discussed, specific questions answered, and preliminary plans for health enhancement made.

Using the Results

Because the GHSI is self-scored, program participants will be able to quickly sense whether certain risk factor areas need attention. It is very important to clarify the meaning of the score totals (usually this information is printed on the inventory) and to emphasize that this assessment primarily is designed to provide a short, general introduction to the personal meaning of risk factors and lifestyle improvement. Participants should be informed that more in-depth assessments (e.g., HRA and WI) are available, but even these are not intended for diagnostic purposes. Participants also should have the opportunity to discuss their results individually or in small group sessions with trained advisors. Usually, one risk factor area can be isolated and discussed, and simple steps for health enhancement can be identified.

The HRA and WI formats necessitate a greater degree of participant and advisor involvement during the feedback session for individuals. One approach to conducting this session is to start off by introducing the meaning of risk factors (those that enhance negative health-related outcomes) and protective factors (those that enhance positive health outcomes, such as consumption of a diet with appropriate fiber content). This step can be followed by a history of the assessment process and then a return of the individual printouts.

The printout for the "Healthier People" HRA in Appendix B provides a person's present risk age, based on how one completed the HRA in comparison with a target risk age. The present risk age reflects appraised risk factors that, when reduced or eliminated, usually yield a lower target risk age. It should be made clear to the participants that the HRA is not a diagnostic tool and thus is not meant to replace health-related examinations. Participants then can be led through the more specific information on the printout, which aligns risk rates (number of deaths in the next ten years per 1,000 population) with common causes of death for one's gender and age, as well as specific risk factors for reduction. This part of the printout enables participants to see the potential effects of their risk reduction efforts (in terms of having a higher potential of reducing the risk related to the listed common causes of death). Additionally, participants can review their desirable weight range, a summary of their present habits that are considered good (for a measure of positive reinforcement), a summary of specific and general risk reduction recommendations, and gender- and age-specific routine preventive services. Thus the three major areas for printout-related discussions with the participants involve (1) making a distinction between present risk age and target risk age, (2) clarifying the alignment of specific risk factors with gender- and age-related common causes of death, and (3) addressing specific next steps that can be taken for risk reduction.

Following these kinds of clarifications, participants can be encouraged to develop a **personal health plan**, which focuses on changes they are able to make. One approach is to have participants write down a risk factor or protective factor to address, ways they will address it (i.e., how to decrease or eliminate the risk factor, or how to maintain or increase a protective factor in their lives), the point at which they will address it, a person who will motivate them to stay on task, and any special considerations (e.g., avoiding situations where the risk factor is encouraged). Examples of changes would be most helpful at this stage. These examples could come from the advisors or from the participants themselves. Also, this may be a good point in the program to offer educational experiences dealing with general risk-reduction issues.

The WI format printouts are quite variable. However, it can be said that general feedback sessions benefit from a clarification of the purpose of the assessment process (particularly noting that they are not diagnostic in nature), an individual or small-group interpretation of the results that personalizes them, and recommendations for steps to take for health enhancement. One WI format also includes a listing of local resources that can be tapped by the participant, a follow-up wellness development process (WDP) for the determination of specific next steps to take, and established reinforcement strategies (McKenzie and Smeltzer, 1997; Gilmore, Dosch, and Hood, 1985). In accomplishing this, the participant works with the individualized data from the printout by using a workbook and through advisor interaction.

Results from HRA and WI formats also can be combined and analyzed for groups (e.g., occupational clusters) and entire communities (see Appendix G). In doing so, composite risk values are provided for groups, which in turn enable planners, managers, and educators to estimate health needs (see Appendix G). As one example of a group analysis, data from HRAs administered to a community group may indicate a very low level of seat-belt usage. The comparison of those data with vehicular accident mortality and injury data may emphasize the need for a seat-belt education effort directed at the assessed target audience.

Reviewing an Example

One of the authors (GDG) was responsible for the development and implementation of a statewide program for interested school health professionals (teachers, school health nurses, counselors, and administrators) to assist them in developing health promotional programming for students and professional colleagues at the school worksite. The program was sponsored by the Wisconsin State School Health Council, which cited among its objectives:

> Program participants will: (1) personally experience the Health Risk Appraisal (HRA) process; (2) review ways in which the Health Risk Appraisal process can be applied in the school setting for student health promotion; and (3) review ways in which the Health Risk Appraisal process can be applied in the school setting for adult health promotion.

This effort was a one-day program, necessitating that the HRAs be mailed to the program participants in advance. The format for the program provided for the following components:

- An overview presentation on HRAs for students and school professionals
- Small-group advising sessions to which the participants were assigned, with continued group discussions during the lunch hour
- An afternoon session describing the results of a statewide school health promotion project that used HRAs
- Presentations addressing how to incorporate HRA formats into the school settings, along with discussions on resource availability at the national and state levels
- A panel discussion to respond to participant questions about the next steps to take personally and professionally

This program included four key ingredients:

- The stimulation of a personal investment and awareness about HRAs by having the program participants take the instrument and discuss the meaning of the results
- Provision of a health promotion example using HRAs that had been conducted and evaluated in another state
- Provision through presentations and handouts of the resource contact persons and agencies at the state and national levels
- Ample opportunities throughout the program for questions and discussion

By the end of the program, each participant had developed a personal health plan for health enhancement using the five components suggested above, as well as a preliminary strategy for next steps with students and colleagues.

Online Resources

Visit http://healtheducation.jbpub.com/gilmore for links to these Web sites.

UW Stevens Point
Lifescan Health Risk Appraisal.

National Wellness Institute
Testwell wellness inventory.

American Heart Association
Coronary Risk Profile/Health Risk Appraisal.
Health risk appraisal based on the Framingham Study.

NASA Occupational Health
Health risk appraisal links.

Healthfinder
Health risk appraisal links.

University of Missouri Health Care
Health risk appraisal.

U.S. Navy
Fleet Health Risk Appraisal.

References

Abby, D. (1986). Worksite Wellness Using the CDC Health Risk Appraisal: Adaption, Implementation, and Evaluation. In *Proceedings of the 21st Annual Meeting of the Society of Prospective Medicine: Equipping the Professional/Protecting the Consumer.* Indianapolis: Society of Prospective Medicine, 46–48.

American Cancer Society. (2002). *Active for Life*. Atlanta, GA.

Beery, W., Schoenbach, V., and Wagner, E. (1986). *Health Risk Appraisal: Methods and Programs with Annotated Bibliography*. Rockville, MD: U.S. Department of Health and Human Services, National Center for Health Services Research and Health Care Technology Assessment.

Gilmore, G. (1979). Planning for Family Wellness. *Health Education*, 10, 12–16.

Gilmore, G., Dosch, M., and Hood, T. (1985). Continuing Evaluation of the La Crosse Wellness Project: Longitudinal and Community-Based Process and Impact Analyses. In *Proceedings of the 20th Annual Meeting of the Society of Prospective Medicine: A Decade of Survival, Past, Present, Future*. Washington, DC: Society of Prospective Medicine, 82–85.

Gilmore, G., Dosch, M., and Hood, T. (1983). *The Development, Implementation and Evaluation of the La Crosse Wellness Project*. Presented at the 19th meeting of the Society of Prospective Medicine, Atlanta, GA.

Gorsky, R. (2003). *Health Risk Assessments (HRAs): New Technologies and Implications*. Elmhurst, IL: HPN Worldwide.

Hall, J., and Zwemer, J. (1979). *Prospective Medicine*. Indianapolis: Methodist Hospital of Indiana.

Hyer, G., and Melby, C. (1985). Health Risk Appraisals: Use and Misuse. *Family and Community Health*, 8, 13–25.

McKenzie, J., and Smeltzer, J. (1997). *Planning, Implementing, and Evaluating Health Promotion Programs*. Boston: Allyn and Bacon.

Moriarty, D. (1986). Health Risk Appraisal for Underserved Populations: An Overview. *In Proceedings of the 21st Annual Meeting of the Society of Prospective Medicine*. Indianapolis: Society of Prospective Medicine.

Powers, S., and Dodd, S. (2003). *Total Fitness and Wellness*. New York: Benjamin Cummings.

Richardson, G. (1986). Health Risk Versus Lifestyle Improvement Instruments. In *Proceedings of the 21st Annual Meeting of the Society of Prospective Medicine: Equipping the Professional/Protecting the Consumer*. Indianapolis: Society of Prospective Medicine.

Rowley, D., Mills, S., Kellum, C., and Avery, B. (1986). Are Current Health Risk Appraisals Suitable for Black Women? In *Proceedings of the 21st Annual Meeting of the Society of Prospective Medicine: Equipping the Professional/Protecting the Consumer*. Indianapolis: Society of Prospective Medicine Publishers, 50–53.

Squire, K., Gilmore, G., Duquette, D., and Riley, D. (2001). The National Content Revalidation of the La Crosse Wellness Inventory as a Part of the La Crosse Wellness Project. *American Journal of Health Education*, 32, 183–188.

U.S. Department of Health and Human Services. (2000). *Healthy People 2010: Understanding and Improving Health*. Washington, DC.

Observational Self-Directed Assessments

Introduction

The benefits of personal observation procedures, primarily designed for the early detection of illness, are demonstrated daily. These are referred to as observational self-directed assessments (OSDAs), because an individual is encouraged to periodically observe various body regions. Several voluntary agencies provide this encouragement through their educational materials. For example, the American Cancer Society has developed a series of assessment procedures for the public as part of its secondary prevention efforts. These include the breast self-examination for women; the testicular self-examination for men; oral assessments for suspicious sensations, lumps, and discolorations; and a total body review for potential skin cancer lesions. This chapter will briefly review these procedures and provide recommendations for appropriate next steps.

Reviewing and Selecting a Strategy

Personal Observation

A personal observation assessment encompasses a variety of physical and mental indicators that provide an individual with a sense of his or her level of well-being. These indicators include body pulse, respiration, temperature, blood pressure, fatigue level, sensory impairment (e.g., headache, ringing in the ears, bloodshot eyes), physical impairment, and mental/emotional response. They range from a high degree of specificity and quantification (such as pulse rate) to the more general awareness of our feelings at a given moment. The intent of the personal review approach is for individuals to be involved in these types of assessment processes regularly on their own. This approach also can assist individuals in having a sense of personal responsibility for their health (Squire, Gilmore, Duquette, and Riley, 2001; USDHHS, 2000; Breslow, 1999; Gilmore, 1979).

As shown by Vickery and Fries (2001), the physical observations can be made quite easily and can complement medical reviews. These two physicians advocate the cultivation of an informed consumer who can undertake certain body observations and utilize specially prepared algorithms indicating what steps to take next. (For example, if a sunburn is experienced with accompanying dizziness or abdominal cramps, the individual is directed through an algorithm to consult a physician. Otherwise, home treatments are recommended for a typical sunburn.) Practical examples of important observations that can be made include owning a thermometer, knowing how to shake it down, and recording the exact temperature, rather than guessing that one has a fever. In observing one's weight, Vickery and Fries (2001) recommend knowing an individual's normal weight and, if weight changes occur, documenting how much and over what period of time. This change-related information combined with a timeline can provide a more accurate picture of key stimuli that encourage greater food consumption. The two physicians identify seven keys to health: exercise, diet and nutrition, not smoking, alcohol moderation, weight control, avoiding injury, and professional prevention. To the last point, Vickery and Fries (2001) state that while most prevention is personal, sometimes professional help is necessary. The following five strategies can therefore be quite important: the checkup or periodic health examination, screening for early problems, early treatment for problems, immunizations and other public health measures, and health risk appraisal.

A clarion call for health promotion was sounded by the former Surgeon General of the United States, C. Everett Koop (1995). Noting that strides had been made in health promotion related to tobacco use over a series of decades (e.g., a decline in smoking by adults in the United States from more than 50% in 1964 to 25% in 1992), Koop observed that "it has jumped back up to 30% with the tobacco companies mounting a new offensive" (p. 760). Additionally, he noted that while many in the nation appeared to be concerned about diet and exercise, "the portion of the population reaping the rewards of that concern is rather small: More than 33% of Americans are overwight," and the plain fact is that "we Americans do a better job of preventive maintenance on our cars than on ourselves" (p. 760). With this perspective in mind, it would be important to encourage individuals to become involved in realistic approaches to health promotion (Mokdad et al., 2004). One aspect we would emphasize are the various observational self-assessments described next in this chapter.

Early Detection Procedures

Breast Self-Examination (BSE)

Breast self-examination was first advocated by the American Cancer Society (ACS) and the National Cancer Institute (NCI) 35 years ago. For women aged 40 years or older, a positive association has been found between the use of BSE in combination with mammography and clinical breast examination and the detection of breast cancer at a more treatable stage. Additionally, the

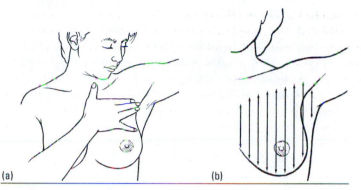

FIGURE 1
How to perform a breast self-examination.
From: Eyre, H., Parie-Lange, D., and Morris, L. (2002). *Informed Decisions: The Complete Book of Cancer Diagnosis, Treatment, and Recovery.* 2nd ed. Atlanta, GA: American Cancer Society, 54. Reprinted by the permission of the American Cancer Society, Inc.

American Cancer Society (2004) recommends that women aged 20–39 should have a clinical breast examination every three years and should perform breast self-examination every month.

With an estimated 215,990 new cases of breast cancer and 40,580 deaths in women in the United States projected for 2004 (second only to lung cancer deaths in females), the ACS continues to recommend BSE as a monthly practice by women 20 years and older (Jemal, Murray, Samuels, et al., 2003; ACS, 2004). The American Cancer Society recommendation for the self-examination is presented in **Figure 1**.

Testicular Self-Examination (TSE)
Emphasis has been placed on the value of males practicing testicular self-examination. Although testicular cancer accounts for only 1% of all cancers in males, it is the most common solid malignancy in men between the ages of 20 and 34 years. In 2003, approximately 7,600 new cases of testicular cancer were expected in the United States, with 400 deaths (Jemal, Murray, Samuels, et al., 2003).

The best time to do a TSE is following a warm shower or bath, when the skin of the scrotum is moist and the testicles are descended away from the body. The following process is used for TSE:

1. Examine each testicle between your thumb and fingers of both hands.
2. Find the collecting structure in the back (the epididymis). Become familiar with how it feels and do not confuse it with a lump.
3. Rolling the testicle gently between the thumb and fingers, feel for lumps.

Testicular self-examinations should be performed once each month.

Skin Cancer Detection (SCD)

More than 1 million cases of skin cancer occur anually, the majority of which are the more highly curable basal cell and squamous cell cancers (ACS, 2004). However, approximately 37,700 of the cases are melanoma in situ, the most serious type of skin cancer (Jemal, Murray, Samuels, et al., 2003). The ACS has estimated that the incidence of melanoma is increasing at a rate of approximately 4% per year. The most common risk factor is excessive exposure to the sun, with chemical exposures representing a distant second place. The American Academy of Dermatology (AAD) has attempted to alert the public to the increasing incidence of skin cancer and has provided a process for monthly self-examination (**Figure 2**).

Oral Review (OR)

The ACS estimated there would be 28,260 new cases of oral cancer in 2004, with 7,230 deaths (ACS, 2004). The risk of oral cancer is twice as high for males as for females, with the greatest frequency in men older than 40 years. Risk factors include smoking, smokeless tobacco use, and excess use of alcohol. A daily review of the mouth region looking for any sores, discolorations, and/or other changes as presented in Appendix F would be advisable for youths and adults.

Preparing for the Assessment

While it is possible for consumers to contact the agencies offering the OSDA literature and request a copy for personal use, these materials usually are offered in conjunction with a program. While dissemination based on individual request distributes the information to a wider audience more quickly, there is less of an opportunity for clarification of the process, demonstration (many times with models), discussion of questions, group brainstorming about how the process can be personally incorporated, and the motivational aspects that a program can offer. We recommend that whenever possible a program opportunity be organized.

It is important to remind individuals who are using these materials that they are not intended to take the place of regularly scheduled examinations or other planned health care visitations (Vickery and Fries, 2001). Instead, these materials are offered in partnership with the health care practitioner in the hope that if a particular symptom* is recognized by the participant, he or she will seek follow-up assessments by the appropriate practitioner.

---

*The term "symptom" is used to denote abnormalities that are detected by the affected individual, as distinguished from "signs," which are observable indications of disease usually detected by a clinician (Rothenberg and Chapman, 2000).

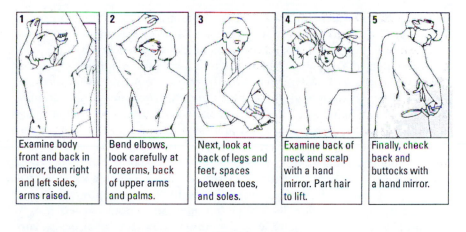

| 1 Examine body front and back in mirror, then right and left sides, arms raised. | 2 Bend elbows, look carefully at forearms, back of upper arms and palms. | 3 Next, look at back of legs and feet, spaces between toes, and soles. | 4 Examine back of neck and scalp with a hand mirror. Part hair to lift. | 5 Finally, check back and buttocks with a hand mirror. |

ABCD Method

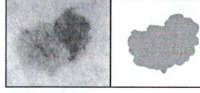

Assymetry One half doesn't match the other half.

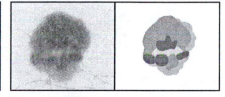

Color The pigmentation is not uniform. Shades of tan, brown and black are present. Dashes of red, white and blue add to the mottled appearance.

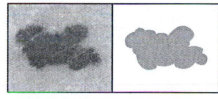

Border Irregularity The edges are ragged, notched or blurred.

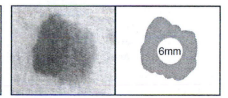

6mm

Diameter Greater than six millimeters (about the size of a pencil eraser). Any growth of a mole should be of concern.

FIGURE 2
Melanoma recognition and periodic self-examination for skin lesion detection. Reprinted with permission from the American Academy of Dermatology. All rights reserved.

Conducting the Assessment

These personal assessments can easily be built into one's lifestyle. They are meant to be quite simple procedures, typically conducted on a monthly basis. For example, BSE and TSE can be conducted monthly following a shower, at the end or beginning of each month. Skin cancer and oral reviews also can be accomplished at those times, or they can be conducted following a routine brushing. The key to any of these procedures is practicing them at a similar time through the year so that a habit is more likely to be formed.

Although health care practitioners can offer patients individualized training in the use of these early detection procedures, time constraints may impede doing this in a routine and in-depth fashion. Group educational activities appear to work quite well in training participants with the basic assessment procedures, as well as providing opportunities for group discussion (particularly so that other questions, concerns, and vantage points can be heard), resource review, and practice with models when appropriate. The use of models with BSE training has been particularly effective in enabling participants to practice the proper palpitation process. It is also possible for appropriately trained non-health care professionals to offer delimited educational experiences to certain target groups (usually with the planning assistance of health care practitioners). It is important to follow guidelines for early detection, such as using the general health detection recommendations offered through the algorithms developed by Vickery and Fries (2001), those in Appendix F, or the specific guidelines in **Figure 3** created by the American Cancer Society.

Using the Results

The key to an effective OSDA early detection procedure is having the participant follow up on a particular symptom or series of symptoms. A person should be encouraged to do so for a variety of reasons:

- With early detection, treatment of disorders such as cancer is usually more successful (Murphy, Lawrence, and Lenhard, 1995).
- One can obtain a more complete understanding of the meaning of the symptom from the health care professional (rather than, for example, remaining in fear of what it "might" mean).
- One can have a sense of being an active participant in his or her health, addressing the health promotion dimension of self-responsibility (Vickery and Fries, 2001).

By the same token, in those instances when no symptoms are detected through the use of these assessment procedures, individuals should be encouraged to view them as positive health-related indicators. In this sense, they can provide some positive reinforcement to the individual, obviously without supplanting the need for routine health-related examinations.

Reviewing an Example

Three national health-related voluntary organizations are joining together for the first time to encourage members of the American public to assess their lifestyle choices and make decisions about reducing their risk of heart disease,

Cancer Site	Population	Test or Procedure	Frequency
Breast	Women, age 20+	Breast self-examination (BSE)	Beginning in their early 20s, women should be told about the benefits and limitations of breast self-examination (BSE). The importance of prompt reporting of any new breast symptoms to a health professional should be emphasized. Women who choose to do BSE should receive instruction and have their technique reviewed on the occasion of a periodic health examination. It is acceptable for women to choose not to do BSE or to do BSE irregularly.
		Clinical breast examination (CBE)	For women in their 20s and 30s, it is recommended that clinical breast examination (CBE) be part of a periodic health examination, preferably at least every three years. Asymptomatic women aged 40 and over should continue to receive a clinical breast examination as part of a periodic health examination, preferably annually.
		Mammography	Begin annual mammography at age 40.*
Colorectal	Men and women, age 50+	Fecal occult blood test (FOBT)†, or	Annual, starting at age 50.
		Flexible sigmoidoscopy, or	Every five years, starting at age 50.
		Fecal occult blood test (FOBT)† and flexible sigmoidoscopy,‡ or	Annual FOBT and flexible sigmoidoscopy every five years, starting at age 50.
		Double contrast barium enema (DCBE), or	DCBE every five years, starting at age 50.
		Colonoscopy	Colonoscopy every 10 years, starting at age 50.
Prostate	Men, age 50+	Digital rectal examination (DRE) and prostate-specific antigen test (PSA)	The PSA test and the DRE should be offered annually, starting at age 50, for men who have a life expectancy of at least 10 years.§
Cervix	Women, age 18+	Pap test	Cervical cancer screening should begin approximately three years after a woman begins having vaginal intercourse, but no later than 21 years of age. Screening should be done every year with conventional Pap tests or every two years using liquid-based Pap tests. At or after age 30, women who have had three normal test results in a row may get screened every two to three years. Women 70 years of age and older who have had three or more normal Pap tests and no abnormal Pap tests in the last 10 years and women who have had a total hysterectomy may choose to stop cervical cancer screening.
Endometrial	Women, at menopause	At the time of menopause, women at average risk should be informed about risks and symptoms of endometrial cancer and strongly encouraged to report any unexpected bleeding or spotting to their physicians.	
Cancer-related check-up	Men and women, age 20+	On the occasion of a periodic health examination, the cancer-related checkup should include examination for cancers of the thyroid, testicles, ovaries, lymph nodes, oral cavity, and skin, as well as health counseling about tobacco, sun exposure, diet and nutrition, risk factors, sexual practices, and environmental and occupational exposures.	

*Beginning at age 40, annual clinical breast examination should be performed prior to mammography.

†FOBT as it is sometimes done in physicians' offices, with the single stool sample collected on a fingertip during a digital rectal examination, is not an adequate substitute for the recommended at-home procedure of collecting two samples from three consecutive specimens. Toilet bowl FOBT tests also are not recommended. In comparison with guaiac-based tests for the detection of occult blood, immunochemical tests are more patient-friendly, and are likely to be equal or better in sensitivity and specificity. There is no justification for repeating FOBT in response to an initial positive finding.

‡Flexible sigmoidoscopy together with FOBT is preferred compared with FOBT or flexible sigmoidoscopy alone.

§Information should be provided to men about the benefits and limitations of testing so that an informed decision about testing can be made with the clinician's assistance.

FIGURE 3
American Cancer Society Recommendations for the Early Detection of Cancer in Average-Risk Asymptomatic People. Source: American Cancer Society's *Cancer Facts and Figures: 2004.* Reprinted with permission.

certain types of cancer, stroke, and type 2 diabetes. The American Cancer Society, American Diabetes Association, and American Heart Association are developing a joint educational and media effort for the spring of 2004, which will focus on risk factor awareness and reduction related to poor diet, obesity, physical inactivity, smoking, and lack of regular medical care (Seffrin, Stevens, and Wheeler, 2003). Along with public service announcements, Web site and toll-free telephone information dissemination efforts, and collaboration with health care organizations to develop screening guidelines, joint initiatives will be developed in local communities. As the representatives of the three organizations have stated, "through an unprecedented and historic collaboration, we will reach an unparalleled number of people with simple, shared messages of awareness and prevention that have enormous potential to save lives" (Seffrin, Stevens, and Wheeler, 2003, p. 1). Clearly, collaboration of this magnitude has the potential not only to apply substantial organizational resources to affect key lifestyle changes, but also to assess and marshal individual and community-based resources throughout the nation for sustainability.

Online Resources

Visit http://healtheducation.jbpub.com/gilmore for links to these Web sites.

Breast Cancer Information Center
Information about breast self-exams, their importance, and links to instructions about how to perform a BSE.

Breast Cancer Agency
Information on breast self-exams.

American Cancer Society
Links with information about how to prevent certain types of cancer.

National Cancer Institute
Information on how to do a skin self-exam.

National Institute of Mental Health
A self-screening test for obsessive-compulsive disorder.

Center for Health and Well-Being, University of Vermont
Information on breast self-exams and testicular self-exams.

References

American Cancer Society. (2004). *Cancer Facts and Figures:* 2004. Atlanta, GA.
American Cancer Society. (2002). *Active for Life.* Atlanta, GA.

Breslow, L. (1999). From Disease Prevention to Health Promotion. *Journal of the American Medical Association*, 281, 1030–1033.

Gilmore, G. (1979). Planning for Family Wellness. *Health Education*, 10, 12–16.

Jemal, A., Murray, T., Samuels, A., Ghafoor, A., Ward, E., and Thun, M. (2003). Cancer Statistics, 2003. *CA: A Cancer Journal for Clinicians*, 53, 5–26.

Koop, C. E. (1995). A Personal Role in Health Care Reform. *American Journal of Public Health*, 85, 759–760.

Mokdad, A., Marks, J., Stroop, D., and Gerberding, J. (2004). Actual Causes of Death in the United States, 2000. *Journal of the American Medical Association*, 291, 1238–1244.

Murphy, G., Lawrence, Jr., W., and Lenhard, Jr., R. (1995). *American Cancer Society Textbook of Clinical Oncology*. Atlanta, GA: American Cancer Society.

Rothenberg, M., and Chapman, C. (2000). *Dictionary of Medical Terms*. Hauppauge, NY: Barrons.

Seffrin, J., Stevens, C., and Wheeler, M. (2003). Joint Communication from the American Cancer Society, American Diabetes Association, and the American Heart Association.

Squire, K., Gilmore, G., Duquette, D., and Riley, D. (2001). The National Content Revalidation of the La Crosse Wellness Inventory as a Part of the La Crosse Wellness Project. *American Journal of Health Education*, 32, 183–188.

U.S. Department of Health and Human Services (USDHHS). (2000). *Healthy People 2010: Understanding and Improving Health*. Washington, DC.

Vickery, D., and Fries, J. (2001). *Take Care of Yourself*. Cambridge, MA: Perseus Books.

Case Studies and a Needs Assessment Simulation

The following case studies are drawn from actual needs assessments in very different settings:

- Internationally based community needs assessment
- Tobacco control assessment
- Assessment with the Hmong population
- Multicounty community needs assessment
- Public health safety assessment
- Worksite prevention survey
- Voluntary agency focus group assessment

These studies provide more detailed examples of needs assessment applications and strategy combinations. In addition to the case studies, a needs assessment simulation game is presented. It provides an opportunity to facilitate a needs assessment experience with a group of people so they can learn by doing.

In addressing the case studies, here are some review considerations.

1. After reading the studies, select one case to study thoroughly.
2. Consider how closely the described situation and/or setting aligns with your present or projected professional responsibilities.
3. Note the particular needs assessment strategy that was used in each instance. Review its appropriateness for the defined target audience. Discuss the pros and cons with a colleague.
4. Determine whether some aspects of the case study might be beneficial to you in your professional responsibilities. What changes would you make?
5. Write down the next steps you could take to assess the needs of a specific target audience or to support the needs assessment efforts of colleagues.

Up in Smoke: An Assessment Process Related to Smoke-Free Restaurant Ordinances in Iowa

Megan Sheffer, M.P.H. and Christopher Squier, Ph.D., D.Sc.
University of Iowa

Introduction

Iowa is a Midwestern state with values and habits that are more conservative than those of the East and West coasts. However, with habits such as smoking, current data indicate that 23.2% of adult Iowans smoke, a figure very close to the national average of 23% (NCHS, 2003). Tobacco use in Iowa results in medical expenditures in excess of $610 million and 4,900 deaths annually (IDPH, 2000). Unfortunately, the response of the state government to the burden of tobacco-related death and disease has been less than adequate, and legislation has usually been obstructed or influenced by the tobacco industry and its surrogates. In 1990, when the General Assembly amended the Smoking Prohibition chapter of the state law to create smoke-free areas in all restaurants seating more than 50, it also added preemption language to ensure that local laws could not be more restrictive than the state code. However, in 2000, the Iowa Assistant Attorney General issued an opinion that the Iowa General Assembly did not preempt local regulation concerning smoking in public places, including restaurants.

Agencies Involved

Iowa City is home to the state's largest university, the University of Iowa, located in Johnson County, Iowa. In 1996, a group of concerned parents, health professionals, and prevention specialists dedicated to reducing tobacco-related death and disease in Johnson County came together as the *Johnson County Tobacco Free Coalition*. In 1999, the group launched a campaign for a smoke-free restaurant ordinance in Iowa City under the acronym of

CAFÉ (Clean Air for Everyone). This approach involved a series of organized educational and awareness activities, community activism, and periodic assessments of community readiness. After several years of planning, activity, and evaluation, a smoke-free dining ordinance was enacted on March 1, 2002, in Iowa City (Iowa City Council, 2002).

Target Groups and Activities

The campaign encompassed a hierarchy of target groups. The major target was the Iowa City Council, the legislative body responsible for enacting proposed ordinances. For an ordinance to be enacted, a majority vote of the City Council is required. Thus it was imperative for CAFÉ to unite agencies and organizations with an interest in health, such as the Johnson County Health Department, American Cancer Society (ACS), University of Iowa, hospitals, and school boards. These groups partnered to provide formal support and were instrumental in the recruitment of active community members to endorse and participate in the clean indoor air campaign. Examples of efforts to raise community awareness and support for the clean indoor air policy during the early campaign stages included entries in the Coralville Fourth of July Parade, booths at the Johnson County Fair and outside local groceries, and meetings with the *Press Citizen* Health Editor. CAFÉ periodically published and distributed a Johnson County smoke-free dining guide.

Assessment

A significant step was the first assessment to measure the readiness of Iowa City residents for a smoke-free restaurant ordinance. Using an independent consulting firm, the ACS commissioned a random survey to assess the needs and readiness of citizens in Iowa City and the adjacent community of Coralville. Findings indicated that the community clearly recognized secondhand smoke as a health risk and overwhelmingly supported a local clean indoor air ordinance (Table 1).

TABLE 1
2000 Iowa City and Coralville Survey on Secondhand Smoke

Percentage of Respondents Who Believe That:	
Secondhand smoke is a personal health risk	68.5%
Separating smokers and nonsmokers does not solve the problem	83.8%
Workers should not have to be exposed to secondhand smoke	79.5%
They prefer restaurants that do not allow smoking inside	67.5%
Other businesses should be smoke-free	88.2%

Process Employed

The widespread community support was utilized in political advocacy efforts. Advocacy activities were aimed at local elected officials through a series of one-on-one meetings and presentations for various groups. The targeted groups consisted of the Iowa City Council, Coralville City Council, Johnson County Board of Supervisors, and Johnson County Board of Health. Throughout the clean indoor air campaign, public forums were held to enable the community to ask questions and express their opinions. CAFÉ also identified specific individuals to serve as spokespeople to represent the group. Extensive use was made of the media via letters, editorial contributions, and interviews with local newspapers, television, and radio.

Outcome

On January 8, 2002, the Iowa City Council approved the clean indoor air ordinance by a 4 to 3 vote. The ordinance went into effect on March 1, 2002, and stipulated that smoking is prohibited in Iowa City restaurants where revenue from food sales exceeds 50% of total gross receipts (Iowa City Council, 2002).

Maintaining the Momentum for Smoke-Free Legislation

Despite the widespread community acceptance demonstrated by the assessment, a major objection raised by local business during the entire campaign was the fear of economic loss should an ordinance be enacted. Such concerns tend to be promoted by the tobacco industry and are always raised as the major reason for cities to avoid smoke-free ordinances despite evidence promoting the contrary position (Dresser, 1999; Glanz and Smith, 1994, 1997; Maroney, Sherwood, and Stubblebine, 1994; Hayslett and Haung, 2000; Sciacca and Ratliff, 1998).

To provide data on the economic impact of the smoke-free ordinance in Iowa City that would be of value to the city in maintaining a smoke-free restaurant ordinance and to other Iowa communities considering such policies, we examined its effect on restaurants in Iowa City. The measure used was restaurant volatility—the ratio between the establishment of new restaurants and the closing of existing ones between 1997 and March 2003. This period takes into account trends five years prior to the passage of the ordinance and one year afterward. As a control, results were compared with data from Coralville, an adjacent city with similar demographics to Iowa City that has never enacted a smoke-free dining ordinance. Historically, Iowa City has had a greater number of restaurants than Coralville (**Figure 1**).

Figure 2 illustrates the net change in the number of Iowa City and Coralville restaurants, expressed as the difference between the relative number

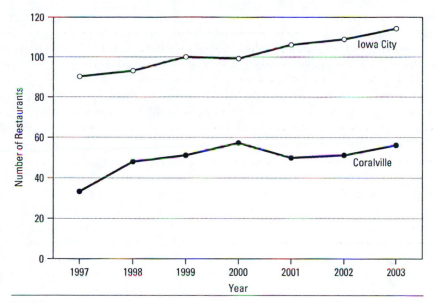

FIGURE 1
Number of Iowa City and Coralville restaurants.

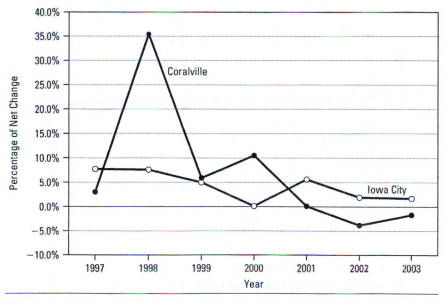

FIGURE 2
Iowa City and Coralville restaurant net change.

(percentage) of restaurants opening and closing. Between 2002 and March 2003, Iowa City showed no net change in the number of restaurants. On the other hand, Coralville, which never enacted a smoke-free restaurant ordinance, experienced an overall loss of restaurants between 2002 and March 2003.

Review of the secondary data (i.e., numbers of restaurants) shows that Iowa City has not seen a dramatic decrease in numbers and that Coralville did not experience the predicted increase in new restaurants despite not having a smoke-free dining ordinance. To fully assess the economic impact of the 2002 Iowa City smoke-free restaurant ordinance on the local restaurant industry, it will be necessary to examine revenue data from Iowa City and Coralville restaurants that are available from the Iowa State Department of Revenue and Finance.

The revenue data will also, indirectly, offer insight into health aspects of the smoke-free restaurant ordinance. Factors such as improved employee health tend to reduce costs because of less absenteeism and lowered health insurance premiums. Similarly, customer satisfaction with smoke-free dining will lead to continued patronage and increased profits.

Postscript

Despite popular support for smoke-free restaurant ordinances in Iowa, a decision of the Iowa Supreme Court on May 7, 2003, rendered such ordinances unconstitutional (JBSCI, 2003). Eight restaurant owners from Ames, financed by Philip Morris, appealed the Iowa District Court's ruling supporting the constitutionality of the Ames smoke-free restaurant ordinance to the Iowa Supreme Court (JBSCI, 2003), where the lower court's decision was not upheld. This ruling represents a major public health setback for smoke-free ordinances in particular and tobacco control in general in the state of Iowa, and it reminds us of the need for constant vigilance by the public health community. Amending the state law on preemption will require a statewide grassroots movement by concerned citizens to advocate for legislation that will, ultimately, lead to the reduction of tobacco-related death and disease. Meanwhile, assessment of the economic effects on the Iowa City smoke-free restaurants can provide important local data to assist citizens and policy makers in drawing up new legislation to protect and enhance the public's health and well-being.

References

Dresser, L. (1999). *Clearing the Air: The Effect of Smoke-Free Ordinances on Restaurant Revenues in Dane County.* Tobacco-Free Wisconsin Coalition, Madison, WI.

Glanz, S., and Smith, L. (1994). The Effect of Ordinances Requiring Smoke-Free Restaurants on Restaurant Sales. *American Journal of Public Health*, 84, 1081–1085.

Glanz, S., and Smith, L. (1997). The Effect of Ordinances Requiring Smoke-Free Restaurants and Bars on Revenue: A Follow Up. *American Journal of Public Health*, 87, 1687–1693.

Hayslett, J., and Haung, P. (2000). *Impact of Clean Indoor Air Ordinances on Restaurant Revenues in Four Texas Cities*. Bureau of Disease, Injury, and Tobacco Prevention. Texas Department of Health.

Iowa City Council. (2002). An Ordinance Amending Title 6 of the City Code by Repealing Chapter 7 Entitled "Smoking in Public Places: and Enacting a New Chapter 7, Entitled "Smoking in Food Establishments." Ordinance Number 02-4000. Iowa City, IA.

Iowa Department of Public Health (IDPH). (2000). *Health Iowans 2010: Tobacco Use*. Retrieved on January 10, 2003, from http://www.idph.state.ia.us/cpp/healthy_iowans_2010.asp.

Judicial Branch in the Supreme Court of Iowa (JBSCI). (2003, May). No. 33/02-0415. Retrieved on September 26, 2003, from http://www.judicial.state.ia.us/supreme/opinions/20030507/02-0415.asp.

Maroney, N., Sherwood, D., and Stubblebine, W. (1994). *The Impact of Tobacco Control Ordinances on Restaurant Revenues in California*. Claremont, CA: Claremont Institute for Economy Policy Studies.

National Center for Health Statistics (NCHS). (2003). *Health, United States, 2003*. Washington, DC: U.S. Department of Health and Human Services.

Sciacca, J. P., and Ratliff, M. I. (1998). Prohibiting Smoking in Restaurants: Effects on Restaurant Sales. *American Journal of Health Promotion*, 12, 176–184.

An Educational Needs Assessment of the Hmong Population in Wisconsin

University of Wisconsin–Extension and University of Wisconsin–La Crosse

Prepared by Donell Kerns, Ph.D., Assistant Director, University of Wisconsin–La Crosse, Office of Continuing Education and Extension

Organizational Overview

The University of Wisconsin (UW) System Board of Regents charges UW-Extension with responsibility for statewide leadership, funding, coordination, and accountability for the extension efforts of the UW System. UW-Extension works to ensure that Wisconsin people have access to the resources of their university system. Through its programming divisions of Cooperative Extension, Broadcasting and Media Innovations, Continuing Education Extension, and its collaborative relationships with the 26 UW universities and colleges, the 72 Wisconsin counties, and countless local, state, and federal agencies and groups, UW-Extension provides a spectrum of lifelong learning opportunities for Wisconsin citizens.

In the fall of 2001, professionals representing Cooperative Extension and Continuing Education from around the state proposed to UW-Extension a project to assess Hmong educational needs. The Hmong, primarily Southeast Asian refugees, came to the United States as a result of the Vietnam War. The latest census figures show that Wisconsin and Minnesota are home to about 45% of the country's Hmong population. Many of the Hmong come from an agrarian society, and many of the older Hmong do not read or speak English.

In the state of Wisconsin the Hmong population has clustered in certain areas and, in some of those locations, represents the largest ethnic minority. From 1990 to 2000, Wisconsin's Hmong population more than doubled, reaching a total of 33,791 residents. These residents have unique educational needs that required identification and clarification if UW-Extension were to better serve those needs.

A needs assessment conducted January through March 2002 included 384 participants in 10 of the top 11 Wisconsin counties with the highest Hmong populations. The needs assessment sought to better understand the Hmong educational needs by focusing on the following areas:

- What challenges and issues are you seeing in your local Hmong community?
- What has successfully worked for your local Hmong community in the past to address these challenges and issues?
- What are the challenges facing Hmong individuals and families?
- What are the challenges facing Hmong businesses and business owners?
- What are some of the educational topics you or others would like to learn more about?
- What would be the best way for you to learn about those topics?
- How and where would you like to learn in your community?
- Are there any additional thoughts you would like to share with us?

In each of the ten geographic areas of Wisconsin, a planning group was established to determine how best to conduct the needs assessment. This case study focuses on the process used in La Crosse County in western Wisconsin.

Needs Assessment Target Group

Approximately 3,500 Hmong live in La Crosse County. The goal of the needs assessment was to include equal male/female representation as well as a representative sampling of different age groups from adolescence through old age. Additionally, there was an effort to include different socioeconomic Hmong groups and those with varying educational backgrounds.

Community and University Planning Group

A planning group was established that included representatives from the Hmong Mutual Assistance Association, La Crosse County Health Department, Family Resources, UW-La Crosse Continuing Education, and UW-Cooperative Extension. Key Hmong individuals from each of the community agencies were essential in the successful planning and completion of the needs assessment.

Needs Assessment Process

The planning committee chose a half-day focus group process utilizing the questions that had been established by the statewide planning committee. All focus group participants were Hmong, and all facilitators and recorders were

Hmong with the exception of one. To gather accurate and complete information, focus groups were created to represent (1) older Hmong women, (2) older Hmong men, (3) adult women, (4) adult men, (5) adolescent girls, and (6) adolescent boys. Hmong planning committee members recruited Hmong men and women for training as facilitators and recorders. The Hmong planning committee members then worked with the facilitators and recorders to identify and make personal contact with potential focus group participants. The planning committee purposefully planned food service, time of day, location of focus groups, and other details to meet the needs of the Hmong community. A small gift was made to each individual who participated in the needs assessment.

Needs Identified

Three major areas of need emerged from the focus group process in La Crosse County:

1. Family Issues
   a. The clash of values in the Westernization of youth versus the tradition of Hmong elders.
   b. Changing gender/role expectations in Western culture versus traditional culture.
   c. Lack of parental understanding of the Western school system that can lead to unrealistic expectations for their children.
   d. Value of early marriage and having children in the traditional culture versus Western value placed on delayed marriage.
   e. Lack of adequate childcare when both parents work.
2. Education
   a. Stereotyping of Hmong limits choices students feel they can make.
   b. Racism in schools ranges from other students calling Hmong students names to teachers thinking that all Hmong should be excellent students.
   c. Very little Hmong culture or history is discussed in schools, making Hmong students feel invisible and undervalued.
   d. There is a need for Hmong language, culture, and history classes to help Hmong students retain their culture and language.
   e. There is a need for more Hmong working in schools as teachers and administrators.
3. Economic
   a. Cultural training is needed in all segments of society to stop discrimination/racism.
   b. There is a need for more Hmong working in city, state, and local agencies and government.
   c. There is a need for more start-up funds for Hmong small businesses.

    d. Existing Hmong businesses need to better market their products and services to the non-Hmong community.
    e. Hmong adults of all ages need more job-search skills.
    f. In general, there is a need for more educational opportunities and funding.

How the Identified Needs Are Being Addressed

At the conclusion of the focus group process, the planning committee met to discuss ways to address the needs that were identified. After some discussion, it was determined that the planning group, with funding from UW-La Crosse Continuing Education, would be best able to immediately address some of the family issues. The Hmong members of the planning group identified a Hmong speaker and invited him to come to La Crosse to offer a workshop for Hmong parents and adolescents. The topics covered included most of the needs identified under the family issues rubric. The program was well attended and very well received, and efforts are under way to create a follow-up program.

Meetings were held with the Small Business Development Center and the Hmong Mutual Assistant Association to determine how those two entities might work together to address the needs identified under economic concerns. Additionally, UW-La Crosse Continuing Education staff met with the Dean of Liberal Studies to explore offering of a Hmong culture and history class as well as a Hmong language class. Both of those classes have now been held on campus, and there are plans to hold a follow-up class for community participants. Continuing Education staff also met with the Director of Educational Studies at UW-La Crosse to discuss the needs assessment and to learn more about an effort now under way to train Hmong individuals as teachers.

Planning to meet the needs addressed is ongoing with vital input from members of the Hmong community. To learn more about the Hmong assessment planning process, the focus groups and the participants, visit the UW-Extension Hmong Task Force Web site: www.uwex.edu/ces/hmong/index.html.

Community Health Development in Mid Glamorgan, Wales

Mid Glamorgan Health Authority, Wales, United Kingdom
Prepared by Elaine Jones, Former Director of Health Promotion

Agency Overview

Mid Glamorgan Health Authority is coterminous with the county of Mid Glamorgan, which lies at the southwestern corner of Wales, United Kingdom. The area was traditionally the focus of mining and other heavy industries, though these have largely been run down during the last 40 years. The population during the 1990s was approximately 550,000, and unemployment rates ranged between 9% and 18%, while 18% of households lacked basic amenities. The county has the highest percentage of deprived population in Wales and is one of the poorest areas of the United Kingdom. The Health Authority commissions all health care for that population, both within the community and in the hospital setting. Health Promotion is part of the Department of Public Health Medicine and operates a county-wide service. The main areas of work focus on the education of professionals, development of healthy alliances, and policy development in both public and private sectors. All services are free or provided on a nonprofit basis.

Mid Glamorgan Health Authority and Family Health Services Authority agreed to invest in the health development approach to health promotion planning in six communities of Mid Glamorgan over a three-year period. The first two projects were to pilot the methodologies and to test the effect that the project would have on future planning in those localities. The objectives of the project follow:

1. To select a set of data that reflects the health promotion needs and priorities of the target community

2. To collect soft and hard data relating to the "health" needs of the community
3. To determine the key individuals, groups, and organizations with the power to affect health in the community
4. To analyze the first two objectives and recommend appropriate health promotion activities that could be carried out in the locality
5. To determine the most appropriate partners in the provision of health promotion activities or services
6. To liaise with representatives from the community to monitor effectiveness and measure outcomes

Target Group

The health development project targeted six communities over a three-year period. Each community was to be self-defining and contain approximately 20,000–30,000 individuals. The choice of community reflected the variety of environments within the county, from coastal holiday resorts to upper valley communities, from more affluent new industrial areas to post–Industrial Revolution deprivation.

Agency Personnel Involved

Initially, each of the two pilot communities was assigned a qualified health promotion specialist as the project coordinator. In the remaining four communities, a health promotion specialist was to be assigned to carry out the needs assessment on two communities over one year.

Needs Assessment Process Employed

The methods used during the project together with an indicator of effectiveness are summarized in **Tables 1 and 2.**

A vital aspect of the project was community feedback. This information was disseminated at two levels. At a formal seminar, the results were publicized and all participants and local health service managers were involved. Less formal feedback to individual groups or individuals who had contributed to the project was carried out by the project workers.

Throughout the project, use was made of local media—notably newspapers and community newsletters—to give information to all residents in the area.

TABLE 1
Sources of Information

Type of Source	Nature of the Information	Purpose
Epidemiology	Death rates, SMR, disease rates, birth rates	Put local priorities against national plans
Social and economic	Employment status, transportation, social status, education, housing	
Local surveys	Planning outlines, employment, education	Identify pockets of specific need
Community members	Expressed needs, opinions, history, desires, views	Identify gatekeepers Identify opportunities for partnerships Identify the natural "flow" of a community Highlight advocates for health
NHS professional groups	Views, opinions, standards	Allow comparison with expressed needs
Cultural history	History and development of the community	Identify potential areas for action that "fit" with the community

TABLE 2
Assessment Processes

Method	Description	Effectiveness
Focus group	Small groups working to a fixed agenda to reach an agreed outcome	Very
Personal interview	One-on-one to an outline set of questions	Very
Observation	Watching the community at all times of the day and night, week and weekend, over the period	Very
Life history	One-on-one with older members of the community to identify trends	Very

TABLE 2
(*Continued*)

Method	Description	Effectiveness
Market research	Opportunistic questioning to a sampling frame	Did not work
Data search	Draw information from existing published data	Most data not available to the local level—of limited use
Media	News items, press releases—before, during, and after	Very

Needs Identified by the Assessment

Project findings in Bargoed and Porthcawl show that the expressed needs of the community are not reflected in the priorities set by national and local plans. A clear example is the almost complete absence of concern about smoking behavior in both communities, even though statistical evidence shows a higher rate of smoking than in the rest of Wales at 32.2%. The main findings are summarized in **Table 3**.

TABLE 3
Assessed Needs

Lifestyle Area	Community Response	Proposed Action
Smoking	No-smoking areas in public houses	Opportunities for local smoking cessation support Increased number of smoke-free places
Alcohol	Help, advice for alcohol misusers Training for professionals Local treatment services Monitor alcohol sales Server training Multi-agency approach	Develop multi-agency, multi-disciplinary substance misuse program
Nutrition	Advice of dietician available in the locality Need consistent messages on diet Local advice and support for people with diabetes	Training for NHS staff Increased availability of fresh fruit and vegetables

(Continued)

TABLE 3
Assessed Needs (*Continued*)

Lifestyle Area	Community Response	Proposed Action
Physical exercise	Promotion of appropriate leisure and recreation services, especially for young people and older people	Creation of alliances with local services Training for leisure service staff Clean up local beaches
Stress	Coping skills training in the community, especially for cardiac rehabilitation Help for careers, unemployed and women	Increased training of NHS staff in stress management
Drug misuse	As for alcohol More advice needed on the use of prescribed medicines	As for alcohol
Healthy sexuality	Include healthy sexuality in family planning clinics	Training for all those involved in education or providing a service
Healthy environment	Dog excrement a problem Derelict buildings Noise Concern about standards of housing Safety issues	Work together with local planners to identify the health implications of actions and eliminate the detrimental effects
Parenting	Need help to deal with behavioral difficulties of children in the family	Training courses

How the Needs Were Addressed in Programming

The project reports included recommendations for future action and suggested a lead agency to take each action forward. The action following the project to date has been positive and encouraging, with agencies outside of the health care field being ready to take on board the findings.

The end of the first phase of the project has coincided with the development of the contract culture in health promotion. The findings of the projects are therefore addressed via contracts the Health Authority has with the local providers of health promotion.

At the local level, the needs assessments are being used as increased leverage to increase funding for health promotion activity.

Educational Needs Assessment

Coulee Region Family Planning Center (currently entitled Options in Reproductive Care), La Crosse, Wisconsin

Prepared by Barbara Becker, Health Educator, and Susan Wabaunsee, Former Director

Agency Overview

Coulee Region Family Planning Center, Inc. (CRFPC), is a private, nonprofit corporation that provides reproductive health care for a five-county area (La Crosse, Richland, Vernon, Monroe, and Crawford counties). Its purpose is to ensure and support the availability of reproductive health care, including family planning services for anyone requesting them. The services include education (contraception, pregnancy, sexually transmitted diseases, decision making), medical services (contraceptive methods, pregnancy testing and counseling, Pap and pelvic exams, STD screening, cervicography), counseling for sexuality concerns, relationship problems, parenting, and referrals to physicians and other local health and community agencies.

The Center was established in 1975. It is governed by a local board of directors. Federal funds provide approximately 50% of the operating budget, with the remaining funds received through client fees and community donations.

A director heads the day-to-day operations of the clinic. An administrative assistant, fiscal manager, accounting assistant, and secretary constitute the remaining administrative staff. In addition, a community educator and a public relations coordinator are on board. Medical services are provided by four nurse practitioners, one clinic nurse, five clinic assistants, and one counselor.

Services are available to anyone, with fees based on each individual's ability to pay. Eighty-five percent of the clients are at or below 150% of the poverty level. Three-fourths of all clients pay some amount based on a sliding fee scale. Services are provided five days a week at the La Crosse office, which also houses the administrative staff. Outreach clinics are held at least once a week in each of the outlying counties. Staff travel as far as 75 miles to provide services to clients in these counties.

Target Group

The target group for this needs assessment consisted of all residents living within the five-county area served by Coulee Region Family Planning Center.

Agency Personnel Involved

A number of agency personnel were involved in this project throughout its development and implementation. It was begun as a project by a preceptee in community health and continued by the community educator, who had the assistance of another community health preceptee. Other personnel assisted in a voluntary capacity.

Needs Assessment Process Employed

The Center began an area educational needs assessment project in La Crosse, Monroe, Vernon, Crawford, and Richland counties. The initial phase of this project began with an informal needs assessment involving five interested people who served as the coordinators in these counties. Each of these people convened a meeting of four to six county residents who had extensive knowledge of the county and were interested in, and knowledgeable about, family planning and related areas. In these meetings, which served as pilots for this project, there were three major focuses. First, the participants identified key issues and problems related to family planning; this activity also helped in the formulation of the question for the nominal group process. Second, participants suggested some possible facilitators for the nominal group process. Third, a list of community groups to contact for the assessment was developed.

From the informal needs assessment, some general ideas were gathered regarding areas of need. People were contacted to serve as facilitators of the nominal group process. A total of 11 volunteer and staff facilitators met for two training sessions conducted by Dr. Gilmore. Besides learning to be facilitators, the trainees provided valuable input into the formulation of the question used in the nominal group process: What are the key issues and problems related to family planning in your county?

A part-time community educator was hired in June and continued with the educational needs assessment project. She began to arrange meetings with various community groups. A total of 252 individuals, representing a variety of community groups, participated in the nominal group process. The actual total numbers of participants for each county were 77 for La Crosse, 55 for Monroe,

48 for Vernon, 42 for Richland, and 30 for Crawford. This represents an almost two-to-one ratio (148:77) for the outreach counties. An attempt was made to maintain an equal ratio of males to females in the age range from 15 to 54 years.

Needs Identified by the Assessment

Using the nominal group process, each participating group came up with a list of concerns. From this list individuals assigned values from 1 to 10 to concerns they thought were most important. The individual numbers for each concern were then added to derive the group value of that concern. Each concern was carefully analyzed and combined with similar concerns listed by other groups to form categories. The values given to each concern were also combined with the values from other groups to get a total value for each category. Twenty-five different categories of needs emerged from the analysis of all the concerns listed by all the groups (**Table 1**). Only 12 of these categories were represented in the top five to six categories for each county. These were listed in order of

TABLE 1
Categories of 25 Perceived Needs, Ranked According to Score Value: Rank (Score Value)

Need Category	La Crosse County	Monroe County	Crawford County	Vernon County	Richland County	Total
Education for Family Living	2 (502)	1 (445)	1 (247)	8 (86)	2 (176)	1 (1,456)
Contraceptive Education	3 (303)	7 (129)	5 (79)	2 (231)	8 (60)	2 (802)
Human Sexuality	1 (540)	14 (30)	10 (15)	10 (71)	4 (124)	3 (780)
Sex Education in Schools	6 (179)	5 (168)	4 (134)	3 (123)	3 (132)	4 (736)
Abuse	16 (60)	4 (173)	6 (74)	5 (118)	1 (213)	5 (638)
Human Sexuality: Adolescent	4 (188)	2 (282)	7 (37)	–	9 (51)	6 (558)
Public Relations	11 (87)	11 (50)	8 (29)	1 (259)	5 (79)	7 (504)
Contraceptive Education: Adolescent	7 (134)	3 (190)	–	4 (119)	12 (35)	8 (478)
Decision Making: Adolescent	8 (114)	6 (143)	3 (152)	13 (29)	16 (25)	9 (463)

(Continued)

TABLE 1
Categories of 25 Perceived Needs, Ranked According to Score Value (*Continued*)

Need Category	La Crosse County	Monroe County	Crawford County	Vernon County	Richland County	Total
Counseling/ Referral Services	14 (71)	12 (44)	2 (164)	7 (91)	14 (29)	10 (399)
Client Education	5 (186)	9 (74)	11 (10)	14 (26)	10 (45)	11 (341)
Moral Issues	10 (96)	–	12 (8)	4 (119)	7 (73)	12 (296)
Decision Making	9 (97)	–	9 (18)	6 (94)	6 (76)	13 (285)
Teenage Pregnancy	12 (85)	13 (35)	–	9 (81)	20 (13)	14 (214)
Availability/ Accessibility	17 (55)	10 (59)	–	12 (56)	11 (37)	15 (207)
Sex Education in Pre/Grade School	13 (74)	14 (30)	12 (8)	–	18 (18)	16 (130)
Legislative Processes/ Social Action	22 (14)	16 (12)	–	11 (66)	15 (26)	17 (118)
Client Education: Adolescent	20 (17)	8 (87)	–	15 (13)	–	18 (117)
Qualified Sex Educators	15 (70)	–	–	–	–	19 (70)
Economic/ Social Motivations	21 (15)	17 (10)	–	16 (5)	13 (34)	20 (64)
Rights of Others	18 (39)	15 (19)	14 (3)	–	–	21 (61)
Abortion Laws/ Funding	23 (10)	–	–	–	17 (20)	22 (30)
Funding of Agency	19 (25)	–	–	–	–	23 (25)
Youth Activities	24 (8)	18 (8)	13 (7)	–	–	25 (23)
Confidentiality	25 (1)	19 (5)	–	–	19 (17)	25 (23)

Note: The numbers outside the parentheses are the rankings of each need category. These were determined by the score values of each category, which are the numbers within the parentheses.

priority for each county (**Table 2**). It is important to remember that the score value given for each category represents the total value given to a specified need—not the number of people who responded. The 25 categories were then combined into 8 general categories according to how the concerns could be addressed. Finally, the total values were added to determine the priority of these general categories (**Table 3**).

TABLE 2
A Summary of the Top Five to Six Priority Needs According to County

Crawford County	
1. Education for Family Living	A need to enhance family structure, communication, and interaction
2. Counseling/Referral Services	A need for more services to deal with abuse, family counseling, and counseling for marital/sexual problems
3. Decision Making: Adolescent	A need to help adolescents develop decision-making skills
4. Contraceptive Education	A need for factual material on birth control of all kinds, including natural family planning and abstinence
5. Abuse	A need for more awareness of and education about rape, child abuse, sexual abuse, incest, and alcohol and other drug abuse
La Crosse County	
1. Human Sexuality	A need to understand and accept one's own sexuality and that of others from a physiological, emotional, social, and spiritual perspective
2. Education for Family Living	A need to enhance family structure, communication, and interaction
3. Contraceptive Education	A need for factual material on birth control of all kinds, including natural family planning and abstinence
4. Human Sexuality: Adolescent	A need to reach the adolescent population with human sexuality education
5. Client Education	A need to offer medical components of human reproduction, particularly contraceptive use, in the clinic setting

(Continued)

TABLE 2
A Summary of the Top Five to Six Priority Needs According to County (*Continued*)

La Crosse County (*Continued*)	
6. Sex Education in Schools	A need to incorporate sex education into the school curriculum
Monroe County	
1. Education for Family Living	A need to enhance family structure, communication, and interaction
2. Human Sexuality: Adolescent	A need to reach the adolescent population with human sexuality education
3. Contraceptive Education	A need to provide adolescents with factual material on birth Adolescent control of all kinds, including natural family planning and abstinence
4. Abuse	A need for awareness of and education about rape, child abuse, sexual abuse, incest, and alcohol and other drug abuse
5. Sex Education in Schools	A need to incorporate sex education into the school curriculum
Richland County	
1. Abuse	A need for more awareness of and education about rape, child abuse, sexual abuse, incest, and alcohol and other drug abuse
2. Education for Family Living	A need to enhance family structure, communication, and interaction
3. Sex Education in Schools	A need to incorporate sex education into the school curriculum
4. Human Sexuality	A need to understand and accept one's own sexuality and that of others from a physiological, emotional, social, and spiritual perspective
5. Public Relations	A need to provide more information about family planning services and improve community relationships
6. Decision Making	A need to help develop decision-making skills

TABLE 2
(*Continued*)

Vernon County	
1. Public Relations	A need to provide more information about family planning services and improve community relationships
2. Contraceptive Education	A need for factual material on birth control of all kinds, including natural family planning and abstinence
3. Sex Education in Schools	A need to incorporate sex education into the school curriculum
4a. Contraceptive Education	A need to provide adolescents with factual material on birth Adolescent control of all kinds, including natural family planning and abstinence
4b. Moral Issues	A need to address concerns related to respect for life and Judeo-Christian standards regarding sexual behaviors
5. Abuse	A need for more awareness of and education about rape, child abuse, sexual abuse, incest, and alcohol and other drug abuse

TABLE 3
Total General Needs Categories of Five-County Areas

I. Community Education	4,822
Education for Family Living	1,456
Contraceptive Education	802
Human Sexuality	780
Human Sexuality: Adolescent	558
Contraceptive Education: Adolescent	478
Decision Making: Adolescent	463
Decision Making	285
II. Services	**1,182**
Counseling/Referral	399
Client Education	341

(*Continued*)

TABLE 3
Total General Needs Categories of Five-County Areas (*Continued*)

II. Services (*Continued*)	1,182
Availability/Accessibility	207
Client Education: Adolescent	117
Qualified Sex Educators	70
Funding of Agency	25
Youth Activities	23
III. School Sex Education	866
Sex Education in Schools	736
Sex Education in Pre/Grade Schools	130
IV. Promotion	568
Economic/Social Motivations	64
V. Moral Issues	296
VI. Legal Issues	232
Legislative Processes/Social Action	118
Rights of Others	61
Abortion Laws/Funding	30
Confidentiality	23
VII. Teenage Pregnancy	214

Note: The numbers after each specific and general need reflect the total value of this category from all five counties.

How the Needs Were Utilized in Programming

Because of the limitations of funding, most of the identified needs were not directly addressed. Instead, the findings were incorporated into long-range planning and translated into yearly goals and objectives. There were two direct responses to the needs assessment. One was an increase in hours for the community educator to respond to the need for more education. Another was a more conscientious and direct approach to marketing the agency to increase the public's awareness of the scope of the services provided.

Some of the findings, such as those related to abuse, were passed on to the appropriate county agencies as indicating a need for services in that county. Involving a wide range of community groups in the nominal group process helped to establish and strengthen links with other community groups and to develop coalitions.

A task force of teachers, social service professionals, and family planning personnel was established to address pregnancy prevention in Monroe County. The task force has organized Systemized Training for Effective Parenting (STEP) programs to tackle the teen pregnancy problem. Choices, a coalition of La Crosse County agencies (CRFPC, YWCA, UW-Extension), was created to expand options for young girls. The focus of Choices is to assist young girls with life planning. The coalition has been a part of a statewide effort as evidenced in a job shadowing program, where girls "shadow" a woman who is working in a career that is of interest to them.

Coulee Region Family Planning Center also increased the presentations in the schools. In addition, family planning staff have been involved in helping the schools refine the Home Economics curriculum to include a course in Human Growth and Development. There also has been an increase in providing educational programs for the community, such as workshops for care providers for developmentally disabled adults and an in-service for teachers on adolescence in the Hmong population. Although funding constraints put limitations on responding to the needs assessment results, many of the requests received seemed to confirm the needs identified by the nominal group process.

Child Auto Safety Restraint Project

City of Milwaukee Health Department, Division of Health Education

Prepared by Robert J. Harris, Jr., Ph.D., Former Supervisor, Division of Health Education, City of Milwaukee Health Department

Agency Overview

The City of Milwaukee Health Department is the official public health agency responsible for protecting and improving the community health within the city. The Health Department provides health screenings, immunizations, health and nutrition education, and treatment for some communicable diseases. Investigations of communicable disease outbreaks and laboratory testing and identification of disease organisms help control disease. The Health Department licenses, inspects, and enforces regulations on a variety of activities and businesses, such as food, weights and measures, sanitation, animals, and the work environment to protect residents from health and safety dangers. The Department's programs are supported by the city property tax allocated by the Mayor and Common Council, plus federal and state money. Most of the services offered by the Department are provided at no cost to city residents.

The Commissioner of Health supervises the activities of the Health Department and is responsible for making Department policies and procedures. All policies and procedures that affect the health of Milwaukee's citizens must be approved by the Mayor and Common Council. The Commissioner is assisted by the Deputy Commissioner, bureau directors, and division supervisors. The Department is divided into five bureaus: Administration, Public Health Nursing, Consumer Protection and Environmental Health, Community Health Services, and Laboratories.

The Division of Health Education conducted the Child Auto Safety Restraint Project. This Division is well equipped to provide effective community-wide health education programs because of its multifaceted approach and multidisciplinary staff. The Division comprises five major sections: Art,

Nutrition, General Program, Special Project, and Clerical. A team of 30 professional, paraprofessional, and clerical staff within these sections conducts community-wide education programs to religious, civic, and social groups, in addition to public and private schools and the workplace. Most critical health subject areas are covered by these educators. The Division also implements the largest special supplemental food program for women, infants, and children (WIC) in Wisconsin, serving more than 7,000 mothers and infants.

Target Group

The population assessed prior to the implementation of the project was persons transporting children in their automobiles.

Agency Personnel Involved

Two public health educators conducted the assessment for the project.

Needs Assessment Process Employed

The City of Milwaukee Health Department, Division of Health Education, conducted a survey of automobile restraint usage in the city. The survey was modeled after a national study conducted by Allen F. Williams of the Insurance Institute for Highway Safety.

Two health educators under the Child Auto Safety Restraint Project were trained in survey observational techniques through a slide program developed by the State of Michigan Office of Highway Safety Planning. Following this training, a survey questionnaire was developed. Nine food-store parking lots were selected encompassing the entire city of Milwaukee, and permission to use them as survey sites was obtained.

The two health educators situated themselves at strategic points in the parking lots and observed vehicles as they entered. Those containing at least one passenger appearing to be younger than five years of age were approached as they came to a stop. Position in vehicle and restraint usage for all passengers were noted. Drivers were asked if they were Milwaukee residents and the age and weight of all young passengers. Only city-resident data were recorded.

Needs Identified by the Assessment

The survey conducted showed that 66% of all observed children younger than 5 years of age were not restrained while riding in automobiles (see **Table 1**). National, state, and local data pointed out the unnecessarily high morbidity and mortality occurring to children involved as passengers in automobile accidents. It was estimated that these injuries and deaths could be reduced by 91% and 78%, respectively, if children were properly restrained in automobiles.

TABLE 1
Child Auto Safety Restraint Project Survey Results: Number of Cases

I. Passengers								
A. Age (years)	<1	1	2	3	4	≤4 Total	5–17	18+
B. Sample size	76	102	135	119	89	521	98	642
II. Restraint Use								
A. None	10	39	106	104	86	345	97	629
1. Child held by adult or youth	27	299	19	9	2	86	0	0
B. Lap belt								
1. Proper use	0	0	0	1	0	1	0	1
2. Improper use	1	1	2	1	0	5	0	0
a. Too loose	0	0	0	0	0	0	0	0
b. Positioned incorrectly	1	1	2	1	0	5	0	0
c. Other	0	0	0	0	0	0	0	0
C. Lap and shoulder								
1. Proper use	0	0	0	0	0	0	1	12
2. Improper use	0	1	0	0	0	1	0	0
a. Too loose	0	0	0	0	0	0	0	0
b. Positioned incorrectly	0	1	0	0	0	1	0	0
c. Shoulder not used	0	0	0	0	0	0	0	0
d. Other	0	0	0	0	0	0	0	0
D. Car seat								
1. Acceptable brand								
a. Proper use	9	10	2	0	0	21		
b. Improper use	19	17	5	2	0	43		
(1) Belt not attached	6	2	2	1	0	11		
(2) Tether not attached	1	1	2	0	0	4		
(3) Improper belt use	0	1	1	0	0	2		

TABLE 1
(Continued)

II. Restraint Use (*Continued*)						
(4) Improper harness use	12	14	5	1	0	30
(5) Infant seat facing forward	3	2	0	0		5
(6) Other	1	1	0	0	0	2
2. Nonacceptable brand	10	5	1	2	1	19
a. Noncar seat	10	1	1	0	0	12
b. Hookover type	0	1	0	1	0	2
c. Old 213 type	0	0	0	0	0	0
d. Other	0	3	0	1	1	5
3. Not used						
Acceptable brand: 16						
Nonacceptable brand: 7						

How the Needs Information Was Utilized in Programming

The needs that were identified by the survey and statistics strongly suggested a lack of awareness and motivation among parents to properly restrain their children in their automobiles. The Division found there was a strong need for a comprehensive education program in the city of Milwaukee to educate parents in (1) how utilizing proper child restraints provided value, (2) which restraints were safe restraints, and (3) where restraints could be bought, rented, or borrowed free of charge. In addition, a community-wide network was needed to provide ongoing education and car seat availability for those in poverty or near poverty. A proposal for a three-year intensive child auto safety restraint project was developed to be submitted to the Wisconsin Department of Transportation's Office for Highway Safety to accomplish these objectives. Information gleaned from the needs assessment was utilized in justifying the funding of this proposal to both the Department of Transportation and the city's Common Council. Without this justification, the proposal would not have been accepted by the Common Council and the extensive existing education network and existing legislation for child restraints would have been seriously delayed in the city.

Worksite Prevention Index Survey*

Sentry Wellness Center
Sentry Insurance, Stevens Point, Wisconsin

Prepared by Ronald J. Cook, PhD†

Organizational Setting

General offices of Sentry Insurance are in Stevens Point, Wisconsin. The company has nearly 4,500 employees, with 2,400 in Stevens Point including 1,700 in the Sentry Home Office (SHO).

Sentry was established in 1904 by a group of Wisconsin hardware retailers to meet the insurance needs of their business association members. Today, Sentry is one of the nation's largest and strongest mutual insurance companies, licensed to operate in all 50 states. It has more than $4.5 billion in assets, a policyholder surplus of more than $1 billion, and annual premiums exceeding

*"The Prevention Index: A Report Card on the Nation's Health" has been prepared each year since 1984 by *Prevention* magazine, Rodale Press, Inc. Permission to reprint the Prevention Index granted by *Prevention* magazine. The Prevention Index was conducted from 1982 to 1996 by the Rodale Press to measure public participation in 21 different preventive health behaviors. "In its early years, the survey was one of the only projects to track public health habits, and it quickly became a recognized source of health information for many government agencies, trade associations, and academic institutions. However, by the late 1980s and early 1990s, numerous other organizations also were taking these measures, and the Index's uniqueness and subsequent value quickly diminished. Consequently, *Prevention* magazine, and its parent company, Rodale Press, Inc., decided to discontinue the work. Nevertheless, Rodale continues to recognize the value that research of this kind can bring to the public discourse on important health issues. For example, it has conducted a six-year tracking study, working with the FDA, on consumer reactions to direct-to-consumer advertising of prescription medicines, and also worked with the FDA to conduct research on consumer use of over-the-counter medicines and dietary supplements. For the past 12 years, it has worked with the Food Marketing Institute to conduct 'Shopping for Health,' a project that measures and tracks how nutrition and health concerns affect food/grocery purchase behaviors. It also continues to conduct research on public understanding and behavior in such specific areas as cancer, heart disease, osteoporosis, and children's health and obesity" (personal communication, Edward Slaughter, Corporate Director for Advertising and Trends Research, Rodale, Inc., November 21, 2003).

†Corporate Manager of Employee Wellness/Health Promotion. A special recognition goes to interns Keith Schultz, University of Wisconsin–Oshkosh; J. Michael Brand, University of Northern Colorado; and E. Patrick Zender, University of Wisconsin–La Crosse, for their assistance on this project.

$1.3 billion. Sentry is rated A+ (superior) by A. M. Best Company, the insurance industry's leading rating authority.

Employee health promotion started at the very first office complex, more than 70 years ago, with the construction of a tennis court. The first wellness center in the 1960s was created when 42 employees started the "Bunker Health Club." They converted a former coal bunker into an exercise area. The professional wellness programming began in 1977, when Sentry moved into its beautiful SHO complex. It includes a physical fitness center with racquetball courts, indoor swimming pool, basketball court, classrooms, and an exercise laboratory with a variety of exercise equipment, plus a Health Services Department.

Wellness Focus

Sentry's wellness philosophy concentrates on areas of health promotion where the individual has a reasonable amount of personal lifestyle control. As recorded in the *Employee Handbook*, it is as follows:

> Sentry has a strong commitment to employee wellness. Employees and their families are encouraged to participate in wellness activities. Each individual is encouraged to accept personal responsibility for his or her health and well-being. On a continuing basis the company strives to increase employee knowledge of the personal benefits derived from a well-balanced lifestyle. We believe wellness fitness and health promotion will help develop a positive mental attitude; improve productivity; reduce turnover; result in less illness; reduce health care cost; and nurture an environment conducive to personal, family, and corporate well-being.

Catalyst for Change

A major medical crisis suffered by the individual, a loved one, or a friend is a key motivator for a change of lifestyle. However, most people are reluctant to change, even when overwhelming medical evidence indicates change would increase longevity and reduce the risk for disease. Esoteric medical knowledge may be a catalyst to some, but it is not a catalyst for change as much as it provides a broad range of activities that focus on involvement by personal choice. Self-empowerment comes with self-responsibility and is best when encapsulated with what has now been called pleasure-based activity. An element of fun and group support for the release from daily work and home pressure is a key focus at Sentry to encourage lifestyle change.

Target Groups

Two of the surveys involved randomly selected employees, while the third was sent to all 2,300 employees at the Stevens Point, Wisconsin, World Headquarters. Available health enhancement activities include those described here.

Program Offerings and Exercise

Exercise programs include a variety of activities. The most popular group exercise classes have been land aerobics, aqua aerobics, water walking, and retiree aqua exercise. These programs are designed to provide an enjoyable group exercise experience within a safe range of intensity based on individual levels of physical conditioning. The classes meet at least two times each week and use group dynamics to encourage regular participation.

The fitness laboratory provides both cardiovascular and strength-and-flexibility conditioning programs. Individuals can participate in a specific program, designed by a personal trainer, to meet their very specific needs or they can join a group program. Body Sculpting is the most popular group program in the fitness laboratory. Pregnancy and Exercise is designed to help women experience a healthy delivery.

Approval of the individual's personal physician is required for participation. Adaptive Exercise is a program of exercises designed by the exerciser's personal physician and completed in the fitness center. The fitness laboratory has a full complement of Nautilus and Universal exercise equipment plus treadmills, stationary bikes, stair-climbing machines, rowing machines, and free weights.

Health Education

The health education effort is ongoing and accomplished by general information in the monthly company newsletter, formal classes, and special events. Smoking cessation classes have been semi-annual events ranging from American Lung Association classes, American Cancer Society classes, hypnotists, self-directed books, tapes, videos, and annual participation in the Great American Smokeout. Any employee and spouse may attend any Health Services–approved stop-smoking program and receive a 50% refund of the cost. If the participant is smoke free 12 months after conclusion of the program, there is an additional refund of 50%.

Nutrition education centers on the company cafeterias. It started in 1977 with fresh-brewed decaffeinated coffee. The next step was the adoption of the American Heart Association's Heart Healthy standards. It has progressed to a Treat Yourself Right (TYR) program that focuses on daily menu selections based on the work of Dr. Dean Ornish and others to provide nutritional and delicious food containing 10–20% calories from fat. Acceptance has been very good. However, the cafeteria does offer the standard menu selections as well. Limiting employee selection or forcing health promotion due to lack of selection has never been part of the Sentry wellness philosophy. Sentry contracts with Aramark for cafeteria services.

Weight management has focused on self-direction and group dynamics. Project TRIM (Team Research on Incentive Motivation) was a team effort designed to use group dynamics to its maximum. The program had good participation but has not been continued. The current emphasis is on proper food selection, exercise, and proper attitude. The classes meet weekly at lunch or at morning breaks for six to eight sessions. A nutritionist is used to tie weight management to the **Treat Yourself Right** programs in the cafeterias.

Stress and time management classes are conducted as part of the Education and Training Department and attended on company time. Wellness classes are taken on personal time. Health Services conducts annual blood-pressure screening where a team travels to the work locations, which has resulted in a high participation rate. Health Services also conducts immunization clinics, self-examination programs, Love Your Back seminars, cardiopulmonary resuscitation (CPR) instruction for first-aid team members, and other programs. Human Resources coordinates semi-annual American Red Cross blood drives.

Recreation

For the past 65 years, the Sentry Insurance Employees' Club has provided social and recreational programming for Sentry employees and their families. The club is run by a volunteer board of directors elected annually by club members. The Sentry Wellness Center Director serves as administrator of all club functions. The largest event is the annual free company picnic attended by 8,000 people. It is held on the picnic grounds of SentryWorld, a championship 18-hole golf course and tennis facility. Other popular programs include the annual Christmas dance, a breakfast with Santa for employee children, and summer-time after-work Tuesday golf. Members pay a fee to participate in most Employee Club programs, although the club subsidizes 20% to 30% of the cost. The company contributes $10 per employee, and there is an annual fee of $4 per employee.

Social and recreational programming has been a plus in the health promotion movement at Sentry. Participants plan and conduct all programs. They set schedules, costs, and food and beverage selections. The company policy on serving alcohol must be adhered to. The policy is stated as follows:

- Sentry wants employees and guests to enjoy themselves at company events. It is expected that behavior will be appropriate for a business-sponsored function.
- The company expects responsible use of alcohol when alcoholic beverages are served at company or Employee Club functions.
- Nonalcoholic beverages are always provided.
- The company expects drivers to be able to operate their vehicles legally and safely. Any amount of alcohol may impair ability to drive safely. If unsure, employees and guests should use the nondrinking designated driver concept or other alternative transportation.

This is a typical Sentry Employees' Club annual calendar of events:

Bus trip to Ice Capades
Winter Family Fun Night
    at Iverson Park
Free indoor ice skating at
    Willett Arena
Company bowling party
Tuesday golf program
Plover River canoe trip
Sentry family picnic at
    SentryWorld

Bus trip to professional football or
    basketball game
Bus trip to concert or theater
Bus trip to Mall of America
Company bingo night
Breakfast with Santa for dependents
Company Christmas party

Family Focus

The Wellness Center's main focus is the Sentry employee. However, spouses, dependents, retirees, and retirees' spouses are all eligible to use the center. Various programs, such as swim lessons, parent–baby and parent–tot aquatic safety, strength training for junior and senior high school students, and retiree exercise are scheduled as time permits. Dependents age 7 and older may swim in the pool while the parent is exercising. Dependents age 15 or older, spouses, retirees and their spouses may use the Wellness Center whenever it is open and enjoy full membership equal to employees.

Healthy employees supported by healthy families are better able to serve customers, the company, the community, and themselves. Wellness has a strong tradition at Sentry and remains an integral part of the company's future.

Organizational Personnel Involved

The Corporate Manager of Employee Wellness/Health Promotion directed the overall effort during the three-year period. He was assisted by the following interns/preceptees: Keith Schultz, University of Wisconsin–Oshkosh; J. Michael Brand, University of Northern Colorado; and E. Patrick Zender, University of Wisconsin–La Crosse.

Assessment Approaches

Healthy Lifestyle Assessment

Sentry Wellness focuses on a healthy lifestyle controlled by each individual. In the initial phase, a health hazard appraisal was administered to a pilot group of employees. The results were used as a basis for program selection. However, the start-up phase focused on employees already making good lifestyle choices. Employees and spouses were encouraged to participate in wellness programs. They were also encouraged to recruit their associates who wanted to make lifestyle changes but were not doing so. The high-risk, hard-sell employees and spouses were encouraged to participate in the wellness programming only when it made sense to them. There was no pressure or guilt placed on the sedentary, overweight, or smoker to join the wellness programs. A wellness newsletter was mailed monthly to all employees as an informational tool outlining classes, providing a health message, and highlighting employees who were participating.

The Prevention Index

The Prevention Index is an annual report on 21 health practices of Americans. The first report was produced in 1984 and each year thereafter by *Prevention* magazine. In essence, it is a report card on the nation's health. The mission of *Prevention* magazine is to provide people with health information and to empower them to act on that knowledge. This theme parallels Sentry's wellness idea. Sentry wants to provide an environment that fosters a supportive climate for employees to make healthful choices. Health is composed of thousands of decisions and actions that each person makes or takes each day. Each person's health is dynamic, and trends toward the positive or negative are based on the daily decisions one makes.

Why the Prevention Index?

The index has national standards with a score that allows each person to compare his or her health behaviors to those for America as a whole. Because it is produced annually by *Prevention* magazine, national trends can be tracked. The index also focuses on health behaviors that are under the control of each person. The questions were developed by experts and have been standardized. The survey is easy to administer and can be self-scored. The index also is void of personal or controversial issues that could inhibit a response.

Prevention Index Survey Results

The Prevention Index Survey was conducted three times over an 18-month period. The first survey, which contained 17 questions, involved a random sample of 100 regular full-time employees listed in the Sentry Home Office phone directory. The purpose of the survey was to gather data on the use of the physical fitness center and assess selected health behavior activities. These health behaviors were compared to national norms. The researcher called randomly selected employees, read the questions, and asked for comments and suggestions on the Sentry Fitness Center or on new programming ideas.

The second survey was part of a master's research project. Information was gathered from 100 randomly selected full-time Stevens Point employees. All names and answers were confidential. All calls were completed in a two-week period. The results of the two phone surveys provided an indication of trends in the Sentry Home Office employee population (see Attachment A).

After the third survey was conducted, the complete Prevention Index, along with a summary of results, was sent to all 2,300 Stevens Point employees, who were encouraged to complete the questionnaire, to self-score their responses, and to compare their scores to the national scores. The employees were instructed to mail the questionnaire to the Sentry Physical Fitness Center. All questionnaires were anonymous. The results of the third survey provided a better comparison to national Prevention Index norms, as all questions were not included in the first two phone surveys. The third survey did not include a section for comments and suggestions for future programming (see Attachment B).

The third survey may be biased because health-oriented employees would be more likely to participate in a self-assessment. The results of the three surveys provided trends on key health behavior. The data were used to evaluate where to place emphasis on health promotion programs. The data provided information on the following factors: smoking, drinking, diet, exercise, weight control, auto safety, home safety, sleep habits, and frequency of dental exams, all having significant impact on personal health of Sentry Home Office people (see **Table 1**).

The survey is a nonthreatening, personal assessment, self-scoring instrument that can be useful to stimulate lifestyle change. It can also be reassuring to the person who practices the health behaviors surveyed. The actions may in and of themselves seem trivial. However, seeing them in print, from a Louis Harris and Associates national survey conducted in 1990, reinforced the need to continue to make a conscious effort to "try a lot" to practice these health behaviors. Since 1993, the national survey has been conducted by Princeton Survey Research Associates.

How the Results Were Utilized

The surveys provided direction for the Sentry Wellness programming in the early 1990s. Sentry, like all organizations thriving today, is preparing for its future challenges by streamlining the employee workforce. However, wellness programming will continue to be provided in a supportive corporate environment. Programming will focus on activities that provide self-empowerment, using management technologies in line with quality-of-life issues. As time demands, issues change, and technological advances indicate, new programs will emerge. For example, the Sentry Walking Club, with more than 450 members, resulted from medical research indicating that daily low-intensity exercise such as walking was very beneficial. The streamlining of the Sentry workforce resulted in longer hours being spent at the desk and thus less leisure time. Most Walking Club members use daily breaks or their lunch

TABLE 1
Preventive Index Survey Results

Health-Promoting Behavior	1990 Prevention Index National Average (%)	August 1989 Sentry Employees (%)	March 1990 Sentry Employees (%)	December 1990 Employees (%)
Do not smoke	72	72	81	85
Avoid smoking in bed	90	NA	NA	98
Wear seat belt	63	79	73	70
Avoid drinking/ driving	81	NA	NA	50
Smoke detector in home	85	96	95	90
Socialize regularly	85	NA	NA	95
Frequent strenuous exercise	35	41	39	25
Drink alcohol moderately	91	81	69	80
Avoid home accidents	80	NA	NA	85
Limit fat in diet	58	76	82	80
Maintain proper weight	24	NA	NA	30
Obey speed limit	54	NA	NA	20
Annual blood-pressure test	84	87	85	88
Control stress	65	60	70	70
Consume fiber	60	62	83	75
Limit cholesterol in diet	50	76	82	70
Adequate vitamins/ minerals	58	58	88	70
Annual dental examination	75	NA	NA	85
Limit sodium in diet	52	70	75	70
Limit sugar in diet	46	44	59	50
7–8 hours sleep/night	64	NA	NA	70

period, which does not impose on their work time or family and social time. Research seems to indicate the best weight management program is self-developed based on nutrition knowledge and self-selection of lifestyle changes. Sentry Weight Management at morning breaks provides nutrition updates, yet does not require a time commitment outside of the work day. Employees develop their own programs and progress at their own pace. As the American workforce ages, chronic health conditions develop, and people become disenchanted with mainstream medicines and embrace nontraditional alternatives, wellness programs must change in tandem. Sentry Wellness is ready to meet these challenges for the mutual benefit of employees, the company, and its customers.

Attachment A

Prevention Index Phone Survey

1. Do you exercise strenuously, sustaining an accelerated heart and pulse rate for at least three times a week? Yes _____ No _____
   (If yes) Do you use the Sentry Fitness Center? Yes _____ No _____
   Do you exercise at home? Yes _____ No _____
   Do you use a different exercise facility? Yes _____ No _____
   (If no) Do you get any recreational activity two or more times per week? Yes _____ No _____
2. Which one of the following statements best applies to you in regard to the amount of stress you are experiencing in your life?
   a. Feel no stress _____; or
   b. Do you feel under great stress at least once per week? _____; or
   c. Do you feel under great stress several days a week? _____; or
   d. Do you feel under great stress almost every day? _____
3. Do you "try a lot" to avoid high-cholesterol foods? Yes _____ No _____
4. Do you "try a lot" to eat enough fiber? Yes _____ No _____
5. Do you "try a lot" to get enough vitamins and minerals? Yes _____ No _____
6. Do you "try a lot" to avoid eating too much fat? Yes _____ No _____
7. Do you "try a lot" to avoid eating too much salt or sodium? Yes _____ No _____
8. Do you "try a lot" to avoid eating too much sugar and sweet food? Yes _____ No _____
9. Do you "try a lot" to get enough calcium? Yes _____ No _____
10. Do you smoke cigarettes? Yes _____ No _____
    (If no) Have you ever been a regular smoker? Yes _____ No _____
    (If yes) What year did you quit?
    Method of quitting: _____

11. Do you drink alcohol in moderation (three-drink maximum when you do drink)? Yes _____ No _____
12. Do you have a blood-pressure reading at least once a year? Yes _____ No _____
13. Do you have a smoke detector in your home? Yes _____ No _____
14. Do you wear seat belts all the time when in the front seat of a car? Yes _____ No _____
15. Do you have any comments, suggestions, or ideas on new programs that you would like to see implemented as part of the employee wellness and health promotion programs?

Attachment B

Prevention Index

The Index Survey

This seventh annual nationwide survey of the American public was commissioned by *Prevention* magazine, published by Rodale Press, as part of its ongoing project known as the Prevention Index. The Prevention Index is an annual measure of the effort Americans are making to prevent accidents and disease and to promote good health and longevity.

To discover which health and safety habits Americans are practicing, Louis Harris and Associates interviewed 1,250 randomly selected adults across the country by telephone. The interviews concentrated on important risk factors and habits believed to influence the long-term morbidity and mortality rates of the American people. Twenty-four key factors have been included in each of the six annual surveys.

The findings clearly revealed areas where the nation was progressing and areas where the nation was standing still or falling behind. With each additional year's data, this series of surveys grows in its power to illuminate a preventive health agenda for the nation.

Once again, the results show that the average adult American practices approximately two-thirds of the 24 behavior items that the series has tracked over the years. The oldest group of Americans is still more likely than the youngest group to practice a majority of the preventive habits, although the gap is closing slowly. There are many areas of improvement, as well as areas of decline, which are reported below.

Alcohol and Drug Use The proportion of Americans who drink moderately or not at all (91%) was higher this year than in any of the previous six surveys. But the differences are not statistically significant and may therefore not be real. However, this improvement is consistent with other reports of declining liquor sales.

Smoking and Tobacco Use If smoking is continuing to decline, the pace of change is too slow to be detected in this survey.

Weight Control There is no evidence that Americans are winning the "battle of the bulge." The proportion of adults who are overweight remains stuck at close to 60%, while 34% weigh at least 10% more than their recommended weight.

Nutrition In the past two years, the public has become more conscious of the need to avoid high-cholesterol foods (up 8%) and fatty foods (up 4%) and of the need to get enough calcium (up 1%).

Exercise The proportion of adults who get strenuous exercise three or more days a week—35%—has not changed. Seventy-six percent reported that they get "regular exercise" either at work or somewhere else.

Stress The proportion of Americans who report that they feel "a great deal of stress" once a week or more often (60%) has not changed significantly.

Regular Medical Tests The proportion of people who say they have their cholesterol levels measured once a year or more often has increased again this year, to 53%. This may be related to the increased number of people who report they are trying not to eat too much fat and cholesterol.

Auto Safety Seat-belt use continues to rise. There is overwhelming public support for mandatory seat-belt laws. Only 18% of Americans oppose them, including only 27% in states without such laws.

Your Prevention Index

To find how you compare to the national average, score your own prevention profile by completing the test provided. Directions are located at the bottom of the test sheet. Compare your score to the Prevention Index scores listed before the test. We also would like to compare Sentry to the national average. Please send your test and score back to Pat Zender, Student Intern—JG4/11.

Prevention Index Scores

1984	61.5	1988	64.8
1985	63.2	1989	65.4
1986	64.1	1990	66.2

Please fill out the adjacent Personal Prevention Profile and return to Pat Zender—JG4/11. Individual scores will remain anonymous.

Your Personal Prevention Profile

The Prevention Index takes stock of the nation's health, but you can score your own prevention profile by taking the following test.

Please carefully check "Yes" or "No" to each of the following questions.

	Yes	No
1. Do you have a blood-pressure reading at least once a year?	☐	☐
2. Do you go to the dentist at least once a year for treatment or a checkup?	☐	☐

Thinking about your personal diet and nutrition, do you "try a lot" to . . .

	Yes	No
3. Avoid eating too much salt or sodium?	☐	☐
4. Avoid eating too much fat?	☐	☐
5. Eat enough fiber from whole grains, cereals, fruits, and vegetables?	☐	☐
6. Avoid eating too many high-cholesterol foods, such as eggs, dairy products, and fatty meats?	☐	☐
7. Get enough vitamins and minerals in foods or in supplements?	☐	☐
8. Avoid getting too much sugar and sweet food?	☐	☐
9. Is your body weight within the recommended range for your sex, height, and bone structure?	☐	☐
10. Do you exercise strenuously (i.e., so you breathe heavily and your heart and pulse rate are accelerated for a period lasting at least 20 minutes) three days or more a week?	☐	☐
11. Do you smoke cigarettes now?	☐	☐
12. Do you consciously take steps to control or reduce stress in your life?	☐	☐
13. Do you usually sleep a total of 7 to 8 hours during each 24-hour day? (If you usually sleep either more or less than this, please mark "no.")	☐	☐
14. Do you socialize with close friends, relatives, or neighbors at least once a week?	☐	☐
15. In general, when you drink alcoholic beverages, do you consume fewer than 14 drinks* per week and fewer than 5 on any single day? (Mark "yes" only if the answer to both parts of this question is "yes." If you never drink at all, also mark "yes.")	☐	☐
16. Do you wear a seat belt all the time when you are in the front seat of a car?	☐	☐
17. Do you drive at or below the speed limit all the time?	☐	☐
18. Do you ever drive after drinking? (If you don't drive or if you don't drink, please mark "no.")	☐	☐

*By a "drink," we mean a drink with a shot of hard liquor, a can or bottle of beer, or a glass of wine.

19. Do you have a smoke detector in your home? ☐ ☐
20. Does anyone in your household smoke in bed? ☐ ☐
21. Do you take any special steps or precautions to avoid ☐ ☐
    accidents in and around your home?

The correct answer for questions 11, 18, and 20 is "no." The correct answer for all the other questions is "yes." Add up your total number of correct responses. Then, divide that number by 21, which tells you the percentage of the 21 Prevention Index behaviors that you practice.

Continuing Oncology Nursing Education Needs

American Cancer Society, Wisconsin Division, Inc., Nursing Education Subcommittee

Prepared by Claudia Bannon*

Agency Overview

The American Cancer Society, Wisconsin Division, Inc., Nursing Education Subcommittee provides consultation on nursing issues, nursing education, and programming to the Division Professional Education Committee. The subcommittee provides learning experiences in oncology nursing to personnel at all levels of nursing practice. Membership of the subcommittee numbers 8 to 15 volunteers who are reappointed annually. Recruitment for these volunteers consists of nurses from institutions, education, and community nursing.

Target Groups and Agency Personnel Involved

Functions of the subcommittee include annually assessing the need for continuing oncology nursing education in the Wisconsin Division, assisting in the planning of local educational programs, and offering courses based on needs assessment. An effort is made to identify the educational needs of the nurse generalist caring for persons with a diagnosis of cancer.

The focus group technique was chosen as an alternative information-gathering process because of the inherent cost of the traditional survey method. Nurses were viewed as a homogeneous group and appropriate for focus group interactions, yielding information, qualitative in nature, with in-depth insights.

---

* Former Director of Patient Services and Rehabilitation/Professional Education, Wisconsin Division, Inc., American Cancer Society. Formerly Assistant Director of Rehabilitation, American Cancer Society, Inc., Atlanta, Georgia.

Focus groups could be repeated in various geographical locations, similar in structure. The focus group technique was felt to be a useful means for developing new programming ideas and detecting problems within existing services. The Nursing Education Subcommittee identified three objectives in developing this project:

- Ascertain specific needs to be addressed in future educational programming
- Determine how existing American Cancer Society programs could be marketed more effectively
- Increase awareness of the American Cancer Society services and resources

Claudia Bannon, Former Assistant Director of Professional Education, and Barbara Sonnen, R.N., member of the Nursing Education Subcommittee, discussed the proposal to use a focus group approach to assess the learning needs of nurses with the Subcommittee membership. It was decided that the priority should be nurses who work in hospitals and who are generalists.

There would be two groups of eight to ten registered nurses each: one group representing staff nurses and one group representing administrative nurses. These groups would be repeated in three locations around Wisconsin. This sample constituted 10% of the targeted audience in these geographical areas, which represents one-fourth of the estimated Wisconsin Division nursing population. Julie Griffie, R.N., was asked to serve as the contact person for each hospital. The hospitals asked to participate in one geographical area, the number of their beds, and the numbers of staff nurses and administrators invited to intend were as follows:

Hospital	Beds	Staff Nurses	Administrative Nurses
Oconomowoc Memorial	156	2	2
Elmbrook Memorial	166	2	2–3
Menomonee Falls Community	208	3	2–3
Waukesha Memorial	405	3	3

Needs Assessment Process

In mid-September, the first of a series of three focus groups took place. So that the focus group leader would not have a bias toward a particular point of view, Subcommittee members were not asked to serve as leaders. Judy Schmude, from Kenosha Memorial Hospital, and Donna Pauley, from Elmbrook Memorial Hospital, were asked to serve as focus group leaders. The sessions were tape recorded and the formal report included verbatim quotations. The nurses invited to attend the meeting received a copy of the following discussion statement:

> We brought you here today to discuss educational efforts for registered nurses in caring for persons with a diagnosis of cancer. What comments do you have to make about this?

To avoid prejudicing their remarks, the nurses did not receive much other information prior to the discussion (or during it). The focus group leaders introduced themselves and asked the nurses to give their names and state their hospitals before beginning their comments. It was announced that the sessions would be tape recorded with a 1.5-hour time limit. The packet of materials presented to the nurses included the following items:

- A Nursing Education Subcommittee purpose statement
- The American Cancer Society Facts and Figures publication
- The Wisconsin Division annual report
- Professional Education Materials list for nurses
- Wisconsin Nursing Education calendar
- An American Cancer Society calling card
- The discussion topic

A coupon for a waiver of the enrollment fee for the Spring Nursing Conference was an award presented to participating nurses at the end of the session. Each nurse was asked to sign a roster of attendance.

A second focus group was held in Appleton, Wisconsin, with four hospitals participating. The third focus group was held in Madison, Wisconsin, with four hospitals participating.

The facilitators listened to the tapes of the focus group sessions separately. Evaluative summaries identified needs through recurrent themes. Differing perspectives were seen in the administrative versus staff roles but were consistent within their own subgroup.

Needs Identified by the Assessment

The following issues were identified:

- Chemotherapy
- Pain management
- Communicating with patients/families/doctors
- Emotional support for nurses: how to handle feelings of guilt, blame, and anger (i.e., "I should have moved faster; how do I handle the family/patient's response to the diagnosis of cancer; and how do I find the time to take care of the patient despite the staffing shortages?")

In addition to these content topics, a number of other issues were discussed and other assessments were made. The staff nurse groups were not as vocal or creative in their suggestions relating to learning needs of nurses in hospitals as were the administrative nurses. It was obvious that the staff nurses had difficulty separating their problems as nurses from the problems of patients and families, and they were somewhat hesitant in making comments. They were not spontaneous. The administrators, on the other hand, seemed to have a broader view, and they did not mention cost of programs as a barrier to participation.

The issues that the staff nurses dealt with related to their own sense of frustration and being able to provide good care for their patients. They were concerned about how to help the patient talk to the nurse, how to help the patient ask for help, and how to help the patient cope after leaving the hospital. The nurses expressed some guilt at the end of their day because they recognized that the emotional needs of patients were not being met. Resources for patients after they leave the hospital formed another issue.

The staff nurses' discussion had a theme of helplessness. Comments about the "politics of the system" were heard. Occasional positive ideas offered during the discussion were helpful at the local level. A local network of support seemed to have evolved in the sessions. The groups realized that within each session they had a great deal of expertise on many of their expressed concerns. It was noted that nurses in community settings are confronted with new technologies before they are educated about them.

Another issue discussed at length was access to educational programs. Administrators indicated that the distance and time were not necessarily problems, and that their willingness to send people to an educational program depended on the topic and the needs of the institution at the time.

The nurses in all of the focus group sessions expressed their continuing commitment to the care of the cancer patient and helped identify problem areas in maintaining quality care in a changing health care system. A letter from the chair of the Nursing Education Subcommittee was sent to each participating hospital expressing thanks for their support of the focus groups and summarizing the information that had been gathered. Two reports were submitted to each hospital: one from the groups represented by their institution, and a final survey report from the three sets of focus groups.

How the Needs Information Was Utilized

The Nursing Education Subcommittee met to discuss follow-up from the needs assessment. It was noted that many resources were accessible, but not utilized by staff nurses:

1. The Oncology Nursing Society has developed and published guidelines and recommendations for nursing education and practice regarding chemotherapy.

2. The American Cancer Society has a catalog of free professional education materials for nurses.
3. Toll-free numbers are available for the public, as well as professionals, to obtain information about cancer care issues.
4. The Wisconsin Cancer Nursing calendar is distributed quarterly by the Wisconsin Division to all institutions with a large number of registered nurses employed. A variety of workshops on cancer nursing are offered every year in the state, and program ideas identified from the focus groups are presented. It was determined that the nurses who participated in the focus groups will be added to the mailing lists for the calendar and future conferences.

The committee decided to meet the expressed needs by providing information to the focus group participants through a direct-mail project. An ad hoc committee was formed to determine what pieces of American Cancer Society literature should be presented. It was decided that three counties in each of the focus group session areas would be included in the mailing project. It was anticipated that 6,000 nurses would be contacted. The initial mailing included a cover letter from the Nursing Education Subcommittee chair; the publication *The American Cancer Society/A Fact Book for the Medical and Related Professions;* the publication *Answering Your Questions about Cancer;* and a response card on which the nurses could request a resource packet of materials from the American Cancer Society. With the initial mailing, 650 nurses returned a response card requesting the resource packet within the next six weeks. The committee discussed whether additional nurses from other areas of Wisconsin should be contacted. It was decided to mail materials to the 650 nurses who requested information on the upcoming Breast Cancer Detection Awareness Project, which was a priority program for the American Cancer Society. A second mailing on the campaign, Women and Smoking, was executed to these same 650 nurses. They have become a continued professional audience for the Nursing Education Subcommittee.

The focus group project successfully addressed the objectives and allowed development for future plans of action. Listening to the tapes gave the committee a different flavor of the learning needs than would be available from a questionnaire. This approach allowed the programmer to hear the concerns of nurses, with their own emotional overtones. It also seemed to be a relatively inexpensive way to obtain information.

The Needs Assessment Simulation Game

Jay V. Schindler, PhD, MPH, CHES
Northrop Grumman Public Health Informatician and IT Consultant, and Project Lead for
Technical and Direct Assistance, Information Resources Management Office at
the Centers for Disease Control and Prevention

Gary D. Gilmore, MPH, PhD, CHES
Professor and Director, Community Health Programs, University of
Wisconsin–La Crosse and University of Wisconsin–Extension

Introduction

For many people, the needs assessment process may seem abstract, difficult, or even a waste of time and energy. The process of collecting valid, representative information about the needs of a target group is not easy—it requires forethought and careful planning. Also, needs assessment might seem redundant for individuals who feel they already understand and empathize with the individuals in the target group. The authors have seen many individuals choose to rely on their own, possibly biased, perceptions of target group members rather than take the time and energy to interact with the actual group members and discover the true needs of the group.

This simulation was designed to give student trainees, health professionals, community organizers, and others a more direct, hands-on experience of conducting a needs assessment. The game can help them appreciate the value of performing a good needs assessment and understand how challenging it can be to get the job done efficiently and effectively. It can be a social laboratory for participants to learn about the factors that make it difficult to convene group representatives, generate helpful survey questions, collect valid data, summarize incomplete information, and more. As an experiential exercise, it provides direct experiences for the participants that a trainer, group facilitator, or educator can discuss during debriefing exercises. It has even proved beneficial to rerun the simulation so that participants can use their new insights and

212

knowledge to improve their strategies the next time through the simulation game.

Like other simulation games, the Needs Assessment Simulation Game asks participants to take on new roles and try out new skills. It is through this practice that the process of needs assessment becomes more realistic and meaningful. The addition of gaming elements (e.g., points for correctly identifying group needs, the limited activities [moves] that each group can make, and the possibility of competition between teams in the simulation) provides additional play elements and motivation that entice group involvement.

Each of the many times the authors have run this simulation, the participants have been able to generate a valuable list of insights and important points about the proper design, implementation, and analysis of a needs assessment. For example, one group discovered that by using two different needs assessment strategies they could "triangulate" their findings and establish confidence in their answers. Sometimes, however, the insights were not always positive. For example, one group discovered that members of another group had decided to lie about their true needs when provided with a questionnaire. Only later did it come out that the trust level toward the first group was extremely low because of how the second group was treated earlier by that first group. Because human nature plays a vital role in needs assessment activities, this simulation game can be helpful in uncovering many interpersonal and cross-cultural facets of human behavior that must be considered when doing needs assessment in the real world.

For those who are interested in using this simulation game in a group setting, the authors suggest you first read through pages A, B, C, and D, and examine the survey and grant application form—the handouts participants receive as they proceed through the simulation game. Once you have a basic idea of the activities participants perform and the progression through the simulation, read through the handouts for the Game Director: Guide for Game Director and Guide for Debriefing the Simulation. Try to imagine your role both as a participant and as the Director for each of the Team Activities listed on page B, for each of the time periods in the simulation game, and during the debriefing.

Although the Needs Assessment Simulation Game activities can be completed in one hour, it can take much more time if you try to prepare the participants with too much detail or provide them too much time to conduct their needs assessment activities. You will know that you're moving at the correct pace if a small percentage of participants do need clarification on the simulation game rules and if most groups feel a bit rushed to complete their final survey form on time.

Don't forget to schedule enough time for the debriefing of the simulation game. This debriefing is your opportunity to bring clarity out of the confusion and to help your participants make explicit what they have experienced and learned. If you cannot conduct the debriefing immediately after the simulation game, have participants jot down their thoughts, feelings, and observations immediately so that they can recall their experiences later when you conduct the debriefing.

You can access additional information as a Director of the simulation activity by going to the following Web site: http://healtheducation. jbpub.com/gilmore. Remember, if questions arise, you always can contact us through the publisher, Jones and Bartlett Publishers. Enjoy the experience!

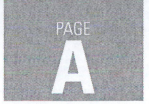
Introduction to Participants

Community interventions and health promotion programs rarely can proceed without first discovering the true needs of the target population. By conducting a needs assessment, the community intervention or health promotion practitioner can ascertain which specific problems are most urgent, which factors might prevent resolution of problems, and who are the most important targets of a community-oriented activity.

This simulation will help you to understand the needs assessment process. Like most other simulations, it has simplified the real-world processes so that you can examine needs assessment within a short period of time. The simulation has, by necessity, left out many of the details that exist in actual needs assessments but has tried to keep intact the real flavor of what occurs. Please keep in mind that most participants will experience some confusion when going through the simulation—that is normal and expected—it happens in the real world of needs assessment, too.

Beginning Activities

Needs assessment activities often require the cooperation and integrated efforts of many people. To help simulate this team effort, the group should form teams of three or four people. Once a team has formed, choose or elect a Team Leader for the duration of the simulation.

[Form a team and choose a Team Leader now before reading further.]

Just as every house in a city has an address, for this simulation every person needs to have an address. The Game Director will come around and tell each Team Leader which street your team members live on. Each team member, including the Team Leader, should then choose a simple address number: 1, 2, 3, and so on, up to the total number of members in your group. Every team member should have a unique address (in fact, every person in the room should have a unique address). For example, if the Game Director tells your Team Leader your four team members all live on Downing Street, your addresses could be 1 Downing Street, 2 Downing Street, 4 Downing Street, and 6 Downing Street.

[Do not read further until all team members have a unique address.]

One method of conducting a needs assessment is by developing, distributing, collecting, and then analyzing a survey composed of pertinent questions. The Game Director has such a survey that should be taken by every person in the group. Your Team Leader should get copies of this survey from the Game Director and take them back to the team. Everyone on the team, including the Team Leader, should then complete these forms *(no names please!)* and return them to the Team Leader.

Team Leader only: Once you have collected all of the completed team surveys (including your own), you have the additional responsibility of collating the results onto one blank form. Simply tally how many responses occurred within your team for each answer to each survey question. When you are finished tallying all of your team's answers, give the tallied survey results and all team member surveys to the Game Director.

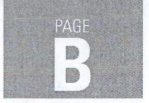

Goal of Teams in Simulation

In brief, your *team goal* is to conduct a needs assessment on all the participants in the simulation—this includes your team and all the other teams in the group. Your team should attempt to find out how *the whole group* would tally up when examining the following topics: (1) demographics—age, (2) seat-belt use, (3) stress level, (4) physical activity, (5) blood-pressure measures, (6) overall health, (7) usual sleeping habits, (8) cigarette smoking habits, and (9) body weight.

Basically, *your team will work to reconstruct the survey data that the Game Director has collected from all of the teams in the room.* All of the other teams are performing the same task. You are restricted as to how you can collect this information, and you have limited time and resources available to collect this information. At the end of your time limit, your team will be given an identical copy of the survey form that each of you completed at the beginning of the simulation. Your team's task will be to provide accurate estimates (or guesses) as to *which* answer was most frequently given for each question and *how many* participants gave that response for the question. Your estimates should be for the *whole group,* not just for your team. The team that comes the closest to matching the correct responses and counts for all the questions is the winning team.

Activities of Teams in Simulation

Your team could conduct a variety of activities to collect the information you need. However, to make this simulation more realistic, your activities are limited to the list that follows. By thinking through the needs assessment strategies listed on page D, you should be able to devise your own methods to collect information. Also, please note that you have limited resources, expressed as MET (Money, Energy, Time) points. For each activity listed your team must subtract MET points from your running total. Once you reach zero

MET points, your team cannot do any other activities. (*Note:* There is no advantage to saving MET points. Consider your MET points to be the budget allocation for your needs assessment—you are expected to spend it all wisely.) Your team begins the game with a total of MET points (e.g., 20 METs).

Team Activities	MET Costs	Comments
Discover the address of the Team Leader of the group.	2 METs/team	Leaders know the most about their own team.
Interview one person in one team until that person says, "No more!"	5 METs/interview	Get information from members of the group.
Get information from the Game Director about one survey question (semi-random element involved).	2 METs/request	Existing records are available, but responses sometimes are not what you wanted or are not easy to use.
Quietly observe one group until the group says, "Leave!" No talking to members.	4 METs/group	Observing members of the target group provides insights.
Make a public announcement in front of the whole group.	8 METs/minute	Using "mass media" can help spread the message.
Mail out your own survey or letter to individuals in another team (return postage guaranteed).	10 METs/5 addresses	Distribute information or forms to the group. Many people use TO: (address) and FROM:.
Ask a consultant (Game Director) for advice about needs assessment.	2 METs/question	Expert consultants can save you time and money.
Rent the Community Hall to a meeting of community members.	10 METs/question	Expert consultants can save you time and money in the long run.
Submit a grant to request more MET points for your organizations.	6 METs to try for 24 METs	Writing a grant takes time, but you can get more resources.

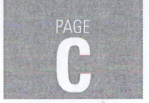

Time Constraints for Your Team in the Simulation

You have limited time to conduct your needs assessment activities. The Game Director will keep you informed of how much time remains. Plan your strategies as efficiently as possible and collect your data using the methods explained earlier. You can use the METs Expenditure Chart to keep track of your 50 remaining METs.

Ending the Simulation

At the end of the simulation time, the Game Director will hand you a copy of the original survey. You will have exactly 10 minutes to fill in the survey as a team. You will now try to estimate what the *majority* responses were to each of the questions on the survey.

For each question in the survey, *circle the one response* that you feel was the most frequently selected response for the participants in the simulation. *Also,* next to the circled response, write in a number that represents the total number of participants you think chose this most popular response to the question. Your completed survey should have one answer circled for each of the questions and your estimate of the total number of people who made that response from the full group of participants. Hand in the completed survey when your team is finished with it.

Each survey will be scored as follows: For each question, if your team has circled the *majority* response, you will receive an initial 20 points. Then, your estimate for the number of total responses will be compared to the actual number as tallied by the Game Director from the original surveys. For each point that your estimate is off from the actual number, 1 point will be deducted from the 20 points initially received for that question. Notice that if you chose the incorrect response you will get 0 (zero) points for that question. Each question is worth a maximum of 20 points.

METs Remaining for Your Team (Strike out the number as you use up the MET point.)
50 49 48 47 46 45 44 43 42 41
40 39 38 37 36 35 34 33 32 31
30 29 28 27 26 25 24 23 22 21
20 19 18 17 16 15 14 13 12 11
10 09 08 07 06 05 04 03 02 01

Activity Bought with METS	Conclusion(s) Based on Activity
1.	
2.	
3.	
4.	
5.	
6.	
7.	
8.	
9.	
10.	

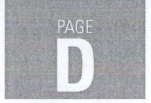
Background Information

Needs assessment can involve many processes, but at a minimum, one should learn about the following major strategies: (1) a key informant strategy, (2) a community survey strategy, (3) a demographic data strategy, (4) a community forum strategy, (5) a focus group strategy, and (6) a participant observation strategy. Each strategy has its own strengths and weaknesses.

Key Informant Strategy

Key informants are individuals who know about the needs of the target group. Although key informants may include actual members of the target group, the key informant strategy often refers to individuals who are *not* members of the target group. For example, if a health professional wanted to learn about the health needs of college students, the professional could talk to doctors or nurses at the student medical center, counselors at the university mental health clinic, physical fitness leaders, or faculty at the university. Each key informant has a unique perspective on the needs of the target group, but the information may be seen as biased or totally subjective. The key informant strategy, however, is relatively simple to perform and can help establish a network of contacts within the community. The typical turnaround time to complete a needs assessment of this type is moderate; the typical cost to do a key informant needs assessment is moderate.

Community Survey Strategy

Go right to the people and ask them what their needs are! This process can be conducted through a mailed-out questionnaire, a telephone survey, or a door-to-door or face-to-face interview process. Nothing beats direct contact with the target group members for accuracy, but problems emerge when you are trying to determine how you will sample your group—do you really want to ask *every* member? Also, do you have enough money and energy to contact a large-enough sample directly? How will you reduce the complexity of collecting, storing, and analyzing your information? Surveys can have a slow turnaround time and a very high cost, but can provide the widest coverage of the target population.

Demographic Data Strategy

Data are being collected about the target group problems and needs through existing programs and census efforts. For example, records exist on the number of arrests due to drinking and driving, the number of cases of sexually transmitted diseases in a county, and the number of female teenagers who became pregnant while in school. Although the data are often available through large data files, and the collected information can be considered fairly unbiased, the demographic data may not have been collected for your specific needs. If a database does exist for your target population, examining the database is a relatively inexpensive way to collect information—if you are given access to it!

Community Forum Strategy

Sometimes it is possible to call a meeting of interested community members to have them help identify the needs within their own community. This tactic can work especially well if the community has some identified leadership, feels competent in changing its own living conditions, and has the time and energy to contribute to such activities. (Of course, many communities do not fit this description.) A local gathering of community members can discuss their needs, modes of intervention, and available resources of personnel, monies, supplies, and other items.

Focus Group Strategy

By bringing together representatives from the target group and then asking pertinent questions, a focus group can help identify the main thoughts and variations within a group. It is important to have a well-prepared set of pertinent questions for your focus group, as well as a set of ground rules so that the group process will be fair to all who are present. This method can be helpful in identifying the breadth and depth of responses to your questions and can be valuable to collect qualitative information. However, if some target group members are reluctant to participate or your group process favors one kind of responder over another, you may obtain biased results.

Participant Observation Strategy

Rather than gathering information about members of the target group as an external or outside contact, you are provided permission to quietly but directly observe and record your perceptions of the target population. As an observer, you can note various aspects of target-group behavior and activities that may be difficult to understand through surveys or other methods of needs assessment. By remaining inconspicuous an assessor can reduce the likelihood of a false or artificial reaction within the target group. However, you must obtain permission from the target group to allow your observing to take place. Although this method can be time-consuming, you may observe activities and interactions that an outsider might not normally be privileged enough to see.

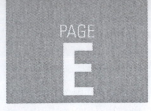

Grant Application Form

Title:

Rationale:

Goals:

Method:

Potential Benefits:

Criteria for Evaluation of Grant Proposal:

Outstanding = 4 Strong = 3 Adequate = 2 Weak = 1 Nonexistent = 0

1. *Title* is direct, descriptive, concise, and comprehensive.
2. *Rationale* provides solid reasoning why proposal should be funded immediately.
3. *Goals* clearly identify targets for achievement associated with project proposal.
4. *Method* clearly and completely specifies the steps needed to reach the goals and see success.
5. *Potential Benefits* identifies beneficial impact on intended audience and future implications.
6. Game Director's perception of the *merit* of the grant proposal concept.

Total Points (If total of evaluation ≥ 15, award total 24 MET points.)

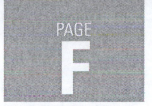
Anonymous Health Survey: The Needs Assessment Game

1. What is your age?
   _____ 20 or younger
   _____ 21 to 30
   _____ 31 to 40
   _____ 41 to 50
   _____ 51 or older

2. How often do you use a seat belt?
   _____ 81–100% of the time
   _____ 61–80% of the time
   _____ 41–60% of the time
   _____ 21–40% of the time
   _____ 0–20% of the time

3. How would you describe the level of stress you have experienced *during the last month?*
   _____ Very high level of stress
   _____ High level of stress
   _____ Average level of stress
   _____ Low level of stress
   _____ Very low level of stress

4. On the average, how often *in one week* do you exercise vigorously enough to sweat?
   _____ less than 1 time per week
   _____ 1 or 2 times per week
   _____ 3 or 4 times per week
   _____ 5 or 6 times per week
   _____ 7 or more times per week

5. Which one of the blood-pressure readings below is used as a cutoff to indicate high blood pressure?

_____ 135/80

_____ 140/80

_____ 140/90

_____ 150/90

_____ 150/95

6. How would you describe your overall health?

_____ Outstanding

_____ Excellent

_____ Good

_____ Fair

_____ Poor

7. On average, how many hours of sleep do you get each night?

_____ 9 or more hours

_____ 8 hours

_____ 7 hours

_____ 6 hours

_____ 5 hours or less

8. Which one of the following items best describes your cigarette smoking habits?

_____ Never smoked cigarettes

_____ Used to smoke, but quit

_____ Smoke less than 1 pack per day

_____ Smoke more than 1 pack, but less than 2 packs per day

_____ Smoke 2 or more packs per day

9. How would you describe your weight?

_____ More than 20% overweight

_____ 10% to 20% overweight

_____ Less than 10% overweight

_____ Less than 10% underweight

_____ More than 10% underweight

General Health Status Inventories

Healthstyle: A Self-Test

All of us want good health. But many of us do not know how to be as healthy as possible. Health experts now describe *lifestyle* as one of the most important factors affecting health. In fact, it is estimated that as many as seven of the ten leading causes of death could be reduced through common-sense changes in lifestyle. That's what this brief test, developed by the Public Health Service, is all about. Its purpose is simply to tell you how well you are doing to stay healthy. The behaviors covered in the test are recommended for most Americans. Some of them may not apply to persons with certain chronic diseases or handicaps, or to pregnant women. Such persons may require special instructions from their physicians.

	Almost Always	Sometimes	Almost Never
Cigarette Smoking If you *never smoke*, enter a score of 10 for this section and go to the next section on *Alcohol and Drugs*.			
1. I avoid smoking cigarettes.	2	1	0
2. I smoke only low-tar and low-nicotine cigarettes *or* I smoke a pipe or cigars.	2	1	0

Smoking Score: _____

Alcohol and Drugs			
1. I avoid drinking alcoholic beverages *or* I drink no more than 1 or 2 drinks a day.	4	1	0
2. I avoid using alcohol or other drugs (especially illegal drugs) as a way of handling stressful situations or the problems in my life.	2	1	0

227

	Almost Always	Sometimes	Almost Never
3. I am careful not to drink alcohol when taking certain medicines (for example, medicine for sleeping, pain, colds, and allergies) or when pregnant.	2	1	0
4. I read and follow the label directions when using prescribed and over-the-counter drugs.	2	1	0

Alcohol and Drugs Score: _____

Eating Habits

	Almost Always	Sometimes	Almost Never
1. I eat a variety of foods each day, such as fruits and vegetables, whole-grain breads and cereals, lean meats, dairy products, dry peas and beans, and nuts and seeds.	4	1	0
2. I limit the amount of fat, saturated fat, and cholesterol I eat (including fat on meats, eggs, butter, cream, shortenings, and organ meats such as liver).	2	1	0
3. I limit the amount of salt I eat by cooking with only small amounts, not adding salt at the table, and avoiding salty snacks.	2	1	0
4. I avoid eating too much sugar (especially frequent snacks of sticky or soft drinks).	2	1	0

Eating Habits Score: _____

Exercise/Fitness

	Almost Always	Sometimes	Almost Never
1. I maintain a desired weight, avoiding overweight and underweight.	3	1	0
2. I do vigorous exercises for 15–30 minutes at least 3 times a week (examples include running, swimming, and brisk walking).	3	1	0
3. I do exercises that enhance my muscle tone for 15–30 minutes at least 3 times a week (examples include yoga and calisthenics).	2	1	0
4. I use part of my leisure time participating in individual, family, or team activities that increase my level of fitness (such as gardening, bowling, golf, and baseball).	2	1	0

Exercise/Fitness Score: _____

	Almost Always	Sometimes	Almost Never
Stress Control			
1. I have a job or do other work that I enjoy.	2	1	0
2. I find it easy to relax and express my feelings freely.	2	1	0
3. I recognize early, and prepare for, events or situations likely to be stressful for me.	2	1	0
4. I have close friends, relatives, or others whom I can talk to about personal matters and call on for help when needed.	2	1	0
5. I participate in group activities (such as church and community organizations) or hobbies that I enjoy.	2	1	0

Stress Control Score: _____

	Almost Always	Sometimes	Almost Never
Safety			
1. I wear a seat belt while riding in a car.	2	1	0
2. I avoid driving while under the influence of alcohol and other drugs.	2	1	0
3. I obey traffic rules and the speed limit when driving.	2	1	0
4. I am careful when using potentially harmful products or substances (such as household cleaners, poisons, and electrical devices).	2	1	0
5. I avoid smoking in bed.	2	1	0

Safety Score: _____

What Your Scores Mean to YOU

Scores of 9 and 10

Excellent! Your answers show that you are aware of the importance of this area to your health. More important, you are putting your knowledge to work for you by practicing good health habits. As long as you continue to do so, this area should not pose a serious health risk. It's likely that you are setting an example for your family and friends to follow. Since you got a very high test score on this part of the test, you may want to consider other areas where your scores indicate room for improvement.

Scores of 6 to 8

Your health practices in this area are good, but there is room for improvement. Look again at the items you answered with a "Sometimes" or "Almost Never."

What changes can you make to improve your score? Even a small change can often help you achieve better health.

Scores of 3 to 5
Your health risks are showing! Would you like more information about the risks you are facing and about why it is important for you to change these behaviors? Perhaps you need help in deciding how to successfully make the changes you desire. In either case, help is available.

Scores of 0 to 2
Obviously, you were concerned enough about your health to take the test, but your answers show that you may be taking serious and unnecessary risks with your health. Perhaps you are not aware of the risks and what to do about them. You can easily get the information and help you need to improve, if you wish. The next step is up to you.

You Can Start Right Now!

In the test you just completed were numerous suggestions to help you reduce your risk of disease and premature death. Here are some of the most significant:

Avoid cigarettes. Cigarette smoking is the single most important preventable cause of illness and early death. It is especially risky for pregnant women and their unborn babies. Persons who stop smoking reduce their risk of getting heart disease and cancer. So if you're a cigarette smoker, think twice about lighting that next cigarette. If you choose to continue smoking, try decreasing the number of cigarettes you smoke and switching to a low-tar and -nicotine brand.

Follow sensible drinking habits. Alcohol produces changes in mood and behavior. Most people who drink are able to control their intake of alcohol and to avoid undesired, and often harmful, effects. Heavy, regular use of alcohol can lead to cirrhosis of the liver, a leading cause of death. Also, statistics clearly show that mixing drinking and driving is often the cause of fatal or crippling accidents. So if you drink, do it wisely and in moderation. *Use care in taking drugs.* Today's greater use of drugs—both legal and illegal—is one of our most serious health risks. Even some drugs prescribed by your doctor can be dangerous if taken when drinking alcohol or before driving. Excessive or continued use of tranquilizers (or "pep pills") can cause physical and mental problems. Using or experimenting with illicit drugs such as marijuana, heroin, cocaine, and PCP may lead to a number of damaging effects or even death.

Eat sensibly. Overweight individuals are at greater risk for diabetes, gallbladder disease, and high blood pressure. So it makes good sense to maintain proper weight. But good eating habits also mean holding down the amount of fat (especially saturated fat), cholesterol, sugar, and salt in your diet. If you must snack, try nibbling on fresh fruits and vegetables. You'll feel better—and look better, too.

Exercise regularly. Almost everyone can benefit from exercise—and there's some form of exercise almost everyone can do. (If you have any doubt, check first with your doctor.) Usually, as little as 15–30 minutes of vigorous exercise three times a week will help you have a healthier heart, eliminate excess weight, tone up sagging muscles, and sleep better. Think how much difference all these improvements could make in the way you feel!

Learn to handle stress. Stress is a normal part of living; everyone faces it to some degree. The causes of stress can be good or bad, desirable or undesirable (such as a promotion on the job or the loss of a spouse). Properly handled, stress need not be a problem. But unhealthy responses to stress—such as driving too fast or erratically, drinking too much, or prolonged anger or grief—can cause a variety of physical and mental problems. Even on a very busy day, find a few minutes to slow down and relax. Talking over a problem with someone you trust can often help you find a satisfactory solution. Learn to distinguish between things that are "worth fighting about" and things that are less important.

Be safety conscious. Think "safety first" at home, at work, at school, at play, and on the highway. Buckle seat belts and obey traffic rules. Keep poisons and weapons out of the reach of children, and keep emergency numbers by your telephone. When the unexpected happens, you'll be prepared.

Where Do You Go from Here?

Start by asking yourself a few frank questions: *Am I really doing all I can to be as healthy as possible? What steps can I take to feel better? Am I willing to begin now?* If you scored low in one or more *sections* of the test, decide what changes you want to make for improvement. You might pick that aspect of your lifestyle where you feel you have the best chance for success and tackle that one first. Once you have improved your score there, go on to other areas.

If you already have tried to change your health habits (to stop smoking or exercise regularly, for example), don't be discouraged if you haven't yet succeeded. The difficulty you have encountered may be due to influences you've never really thought about—such as advertising—or to a lack of support and encouragement. Understanding these influences is an important step toward changing the way they affect you.

There's Help Available. In addition to personal actions you can take on your own, there are community programs and groups (such as the YMCA or the local chapter of the American Heart Association) that can assist you and your family to make the changes you want to make. If you want to know more about these groups or about health risks, contact your local health department or the National Health Information Clearinghouse. There's a lot you can do to stay healthy or to improve your health—and there are organizations that can help you. Start a new HEALTHSTYLE today!

Source: Single copies of "Healthstyle" are available at no charge to Wisconsin residents through the Wisconsin Clearinghouse for Prevention Resources in Madison, Wisconsin, by calling 608-262-9157. Used with the permission of the Wisconsin Clearinghouse for Prevention Resources. Other sources of "Healthstyle" include:

- The University of Florida Cooperative Extension: http://edis.at.ufl.edu/HE778
- The Centers for Disease Control and Prevention and Clemson University: http://www.cdc.gov/nasd/docs/d001201-d001300/d001245/d001245.html.

Living Smart Quiz

Are you living smart? Check "Yes" or "No" next to each question, then keep reading to see how you can keep living smart!

Yes	No	
☐	☐	1. I eat at least five servings of vegetables and fruits every day.
☐	☐	2. I eat at least six servings of bread, rice, pasta, and cereal every day.
☐	☐	3. I drink reduced-fat or fat-free milk and yogurt, and seldom eat high-fat cheeses.
☐	☐	4. I rarely eat high-fat meat like bacon, hot dogs, sausage, steak, or ground beef.
☐	☐	5. I take it easy on high-fat baked goods such as pies, cakes, cookies, sweet rolls, and doughnuts.
☐	☐	6. I rarely add butter, margarine, oil, sour cream, or mayonnaise to foods when I'm cooking or at the table.
☐	☐	7. I rarely (less than twice a week) eat fried foods.
☐	☐	8. I try to maintain a healthy weight.
☐	☐	9. I am physically active for at least 30 minutes on most days of the week.
☐	☐	10. I usually take the stairs instead of waiting for an elevator.
☐	☐	11. I try to spend most of my free time being active, instead of watching television or sitting at the computer.
☐	☐	12. I never, or only occasionally, drink alcohol.

How do you rate?

0–4 YES Answers: Diet Alert!
Your diet is probably too high in fat and too low in plant foods like vegetables, fruits, and grains. You may want to take a look at your eating habits and find ways to make some changes. Need to increase your vegetables and fruits? Trying to watch your fat?

4–8 YES Answers: Not Bad! You're Halfway There!
You still have a way to go. Look at your NO answers to help you decide which areas of your diet need to be improved, or whether your physical activity level should be increased.

9–12 YES Answers: Good For You! You're Living Smart!
Keep up the good habits and keep looking for ways to improve.

Source: American Cancer Society's *Living Smart: The American Cancer Society's Guide to Eating Healthy and Being Active.* Reprinted with permission.

Health Risk Appraisals

Bob Gorsky, PhD

Health Risk Assessments (HRAs): New Technologies and Implications

Shift from Paper-Based to Technology-Based HRAs

Paper-based HRAs were the standard for about 25 years until the late 1990s, when the electronics era began fostering technology innovations (and additional options) in the design, implementation, and application of HRAs as a population health management tool.

About 1998, new HRA innovations began to appear (in the HRA industry) as an option for employers, health plans, and other groups. Examples include the following:

- In late 1998, HPN WorldWide and Wellness, Inc., released a next-generation HRA called the Health Power Profile (HPP) using Palm computing (a.k.a. personal digital assistants/PDA) technology to capture the data in conjunction with or independent of health screenings.
- Between 1998 and 2000, Staywell, Inc., and other vendors released Internet versions of their conventional paper-based HRAs.

Palm-Technology HRAs

To date, more than 200,000 people have used Palm-based HRAs. Here are some noteworthy findings:

- Completion time is cut by 60% or more (versus paper), taking five minutes to complete 40–50 questions

- Participation rates nearly doubled
- No questions are skipped—better data capture
- Money is saved from paper questionnaires not being needed and related costs, scanning time, and postage
- Participants are attracted to the technology regardless of age, gender, education level, or ethnicity
- Fewer than ten people asked for a paper version
- No Palm devices disappeared
- Customization of questions was easier, faster, and less costly

These findings apply whether the HPP was done in conjunction with or independent of an early detection screening (e.g., blood pressure, cholesterol, and other clinical tests).

When done in conjunction with voluntary worksite early detection screenings, significantly more (90–97%) screening participants completed the Palm technology-based HRA as compared to the paper-based HRA offered in previous years (47–55%).

Internet-Based HRAs

Our work with groups who have tried Internet-based HRAs has yielded the following observations:

- Participation rates are far lower than expected. In fact, they are lower than completion rates of the same paper-based HRAs done in previous years.
- It is not uncommon for users completing the online HRA to stop and not finish it for any of multiple reasons—slow computer, dial-up modem, ISP (e.g., AOL) terminating the session, interruptions at work or home.
- Employee communications regarding the Internet-based HRA were much more involved than anticipated and still yielded less than desirable participation rates.
- When done in conjunction with worksite early detection screenings, significantly fewer screening participants completed the Internet-based HRA (as compared to the paper-based HRA in previous years).

Discussion

The pros and cons of electronic HRAs appear to be specific to the type of technology used and setting (e.g., worksite).

Palm-based HRAs appear to dramatically improve HRA participation rates, data capture, efficiencies, and cost-effectiveness. The current form and/or implementation methods of Internet-based HRAs appear to have many disadvantages (listed above).

Regardless of the technology platform, there are other variables (common to any option) that can influence HRA participation rates, such as the following:

- Promotional efforts and communications
- Design of personal reports
- Completion incentives
- User interface—paper, palm, screen, layout
- Convenience—time during work or during screening to complete, completion time
- Access—computer, high-speed line (broadband)

Regarding access, Internet-based and paper-based HRAs may be more amenable to employees who cannot attend a worksite screening (e.g., remote employees), but the findings suggest caution before considering them as a primary option (see next page).

Before full confidence can be placed in Internet-based HRAs, further exploration of the best design and implementation methods appears critically needed to increase participation rates to acceptable levels of success.

As always with any HRA, no HRA (regardless of platform) should be done without serious committment to linking to existing resources (e.g., health screenings, follow-up information and resources, training) and/or adding appropriate support resources to help participants begin to reduce and better manage identified risks.

Conclusions and Best Practice Recommendations

From research and field experience over the past 25 years (including the past five technology platform–related years), our conclusions (assuming all other variables are equal) are as follows:

1. Palm-based HRAs generate the best participation rates.
2. Paper-based HRAs generate moderate participation rates.
3. Internet HRAs yield the lowest participation rates.

Based on findings to date, we recommend the following as HRA best practices:

A. Use Palm-based HRAs especially in conjunction with worksite implementation methods, with or without screenings.
B. Use paper-based HRAs where Palm-based HRAs are not feasible and/or for those individuals less inclined toward technology-based HRAs.
C. Carefully review Internet-based HRAs and implementation methods to avoid low participation rates and program failure (see D and E below).
D. Consider B or C as feasible options for hard-to-reach individuals (e.g., small worksites, working at home).

E. If C is being considered as the primary population-wide method, pilot test the proposed approach before major commitments and resources are applied.

F. To maximize participation success, time, data capture, and cost efficiencies, implement HRAs and core health screenings at the same time—using option A as the primary HRA method, B as a back-up, and C when appropriate.

For More Information:

1. U.S. Preventive Services Task Force (1996). *A Guide to Clinical Preventive Services,* 2nd ed. Baltimore: Williams & Wilkins.
2. Gorsky, Larson. (2002). *Best Practices: Health Risk Management and Loss Control,* 3rd ed. Elmhurst, IL: HPN WorldWide.
3. www.hpn.com/screenings.html.
4. Bob Gorsky, Ph.D.: bobgorsky@hpn.com
   630.941.9030

Note: More than 50 employers (e.g., businesses, government, schools) using the technology platforms discussed with more than 200,000 employees across more than 400 worksites throughout the United States were considered in this update.

Source: Used with permission: HPN WorldWide, Inc. www.hpn.com.

C

La Crosse Wellness Project

Preface

Welcome to the Wellness Development Process of the La Crosse Wellness Project (LWP). Earlier you completed the La Crosse Wellness Inventory, which was the **Assessment** stage. Now you have the opportunity to go through the **Intervention** and **Reinforcement** stages of wellness. In these stages, you will examine your current level of wellness and establish a process for wellness enhancement in your life.

There are several points that we would like to make before you continue. Please notice that we have made every effort in this project to stay away from establishing the kind of scoring system that forces you to compare yourself with others. While we believe that "comparing ourselves to others" is **one** way of valuing our lives, we also believe that people should learn how to value themselves. This means comparing yourself with yourself, rather than constantly comparing yourself to the expectations of society. As a result, we have designed an inventory that encourages you to assess yourself and then to make decisions about **your** assessment. This provides you with the basis to make some plans for your lifestyle choices.

Your potential for an improved lifestyle corresponds to your investment in reading the Wellness Development Process booklet and your investment in understanding the process. We recognize that this booklet is lengthy. Its structure provides you with educational and conceptual information on the left side and a worksheet to the right. We highly recommend that you take the time to read the information on the left before completing the worksheet to the right.

The Wellness Development Process, contained in this booklet, consists of four sections:

1. Establishing a Wellness Area for Enhancement
2. Identifying Wellness Outcomes
3. Establishing Wellness Activities
4. Working Toward Personal Enhancement

Their order and content are designed to foster specific understanding of how to make changes in your life. The purpose of the LWP is to help you learn how to:

1. Assess your life
2. Select areas for enhancement
3. Establish activities for enhancement
4. Establish rewards for enhancement

Wellness involves a lifelong learning process in which health-related decisions are made to maximize your health promotion potential. Health promotion is a way of life and the responsibility belongs to each of us.

You will get out of this development process what you choose to put into it.

Margaret F. Dosch
Gary D. Gilmore
Thomas L. Hood

Steering Committee Members
for the La Crosse Wellness Project

Introduction

What Do You Most Want from Life?

If someone were to ask you this question, how would you respond? Obviously, the answers that people give to this question are numerous and diverse; yet, there appears to be a common theme that underlies the answer of most people. At a more basic level, it appears that what most people want from life is "to be happy." Most of the things that we work for in life—"to get an education," "develop relationships," "earn money," "be important," etc.—are all achieved to create some form of happiness.

How Do We Attain Happiness?

Answers are equally different for this question. How or what creates happiness is different for different people. Yet, once again, we find common factors that help to create happiness. Two such factors are (1) achieving some level of success in what we attempt, and (2) feeling like we are able to have an impact on our lives so as not to feel overwhelmed.

Consider: "How will you **learn** how to increase your chance of success, to feel good about yourself, and to make choices that will have an impact on your life?" This question relates to the heart of the La Crosse Wellness Project, which is to help you as an individual to (1) understand how you can become more aware of your present lifestyle, (2) design a plan for your own lifestyle changes, and (3) overall, improve your feelings about yourself.

Wellness is **not** sitting around waiting for the world to provide you with what you want, and complaining when it does not happen. Wellness **is** an active process. The process includes:

1. Accepting yourself as human, identifying your strengths and weaknesses, learning to accept those that you cannot change, and establishing a process for changing those for which you can be more responsible.
2. Reducing your world into workable outcomes and activities.
3. Taking ownership and responsibility for what you believe in and for your own decisions.
4. Perceiving yourself as able to make changes and not allowing yourself to be overwhelmed by the many small problems of life or the major problems of life to the point of becoming frustrated.
5. Seeing the big picture of life.
6. Learning how to strive for excellence in life rather than trying to be perfect.
7. Establishing expectations, outcomes, and activities that are achievable, yet challenging, and doing this in such a way that you do not set yourself up for failure.
8. Not letting yourself rationalize the difficulties of life.
9. Seeing yourself as human, being made up of many parts that include feelings, beliefs, and behaviors, and recognizing that you cannot be perfect in all of these areas and that this is OK.
10. Taking areas of your life you have identified for change and developing activities to achieve that change.
11. Addressing positive and negative issues in your life.

Wellness is all of these and more. You are probably able to add more statements to this list. The purpose of the La Crosse Wellness Project is to get you thinking about wellness and to recognize that you, as an individual, have a terrific amount of potential to improve your own life and to affect your own sense of happiness.

The process that follows is a method to reduce large areas into workable units. Three factors are used in reducing a large area: need, ability, and desire. These interrelated factors are vital to success.

1. Establishing a Wellness Area for Enhancement

Educational Module

The worksheet on the right page is designed to guide you through a process that enables you to narrow down the nine areas of wellness to the one that you now wish to attempt to change. (A common error that prevents our effectively changing our lives is that we see problems as "too big" because we don't know how to narrow them down.)

Enhancement means reducing or eliminating unhealthy actions and/or maintaining or improving healthy actions in each wellness area.

A unique educational concept in the La Crosse Wellness Project (LWP) is:

That we too frequently compare ourselves to others and do not look into ourselves. We do this by comparing our "scores" with others' "scores" or by comparing ourselves with what is "normal." Too frequently, this does not allow us to find value in the positive things we do because they seem to be "not enough." This project encourages you to focus on yourself and to give yourself credit for all the positives you create in your lifestyle, even when you may see a need to do more. Your ability to feel good about yourself and to see yourself as being able to change is related to your ability to acknowledge positive behaviors, even when you recognize you have improvements to make.

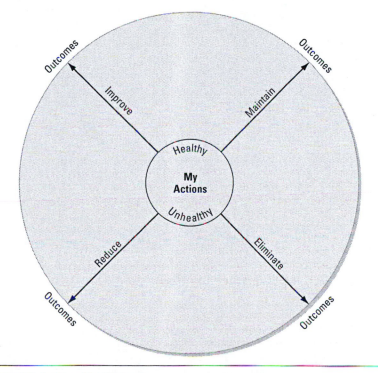

Enhancement Moving Toward Total Wellness
Enhancement means reducing or eliminating unhealthy actions in your life, and/or maintaining or improving healthy actions in your life. As you prepare to take your action steps, examine the figure so that you can visualize the enhancement process. Used with permission from the La Crosse Wellness Project.

Available Health Risk Appraisals and Wellness Inventories

Title	Scoring Process	Description	URL	Contact
La Crosse Wellness Project	Computer	Emphasizes current levels of wellness with follow-up materials for planned change and reinforcement.	Dr. Gilmore: gilmore.gary@uwlax.edu	La Crosse Wellness Project, 203 Mitchell Hall University of Wisconsin–La Crosse, La Crosse, WI 54601 Telephone: (608) 785-8162
Lifescan	Computer	Emphasizes physical activity, drug usage, driving habits, cholesterol level, medical history, and women's health issues.	http://wellness.uwsp.edu/Health_Service/Services/lifescan.htm	Lifestyle Improvement Systems, 718 Linwood Avenue, Stevens Point, WI 54481 Telephone: (715) 345-1735
Personal Wellness Profile	Computer	Addresses worksite wellness through assessments of coronary and cancer risk, fitness, lung function, body composition, nutrition, tobacco and alcohol use, and blood pressure.	http://www.wellsource.com/products/web.htm	Wellsource, P.O. Box 569, Clackamas, OR Telephone: (503) 656-7446

(Continued)

Title	Scoring Process	Description	URL	Contact
QuickCheck	Computer	The Wellsource QuickCheck Online Assessment Suite offers information needed to recognize possible health risks. It provides instruction on how to reach optimal health.	http://www.wellsource.com/products/web.htm	Wellsource, P.O. Box 569, Clackamas, OR Telephone: (503) 656-7446
Testwell (HLQ or HRA)	Computer	Measures strength in social, occupational, spiritual, physical, intellectual, and emotional dimensions of wellness.	http://www.testwell.org/	National Wellness Institute, 1300 College Ct., P.O. Box 827, Stevens Point, WI 54481 Telephone: (715) 342-2969
IHRA Online	Computer	Analyzes medical factors and lifestyle choices. It is a customized, programmed,	http://www.hraonline.com/	CPM Corporate Offices and Technology Center, 6720 Frank Lloyd Wright Ave.,

		mortality-based instrument that can estimate participants' longevity.	Ste. 200, Middleton, WI 53562 Telephone: (608) 831-7880 (800) 332-2631 Fax: (608) 831-7889
You First Health Risk Assessment	Computer	Includes major risk factors related to lifestyle, including wellness, exercise, nutrition, smoking, alcohol use, weight, cholesterol, blood pressure, back pain, vehicle safety, stress, depression, and cancer.	http://www.youfirst.com/	Customer Service Representative, You First, Bridgewater, NJ Telephone: (800) 561-3261

E

Community Capacity Assessment Inventory

UNITED NEIGHBORS
Capacity Survey

What would you say are some of the best things about our neighborhood?

_____

_____

Why did you choose to live here?

_____

_____

What are some thing that you would like to do to improve the neighborhood?

_____

_____

Have you ever participated in any of the following activities?

_____ Boy Scouts/Girl Scouts
_____ Church fundraisers
_____ Bingo
_____ PTA or school associations
_____ Sports teams
_____ Camp trips or field trips
_____ Political campaigns
_____ Neighborhood associations
_____ Rummage sales or yard sales
_____ Church suppers
_____ Tutoring
_____ 4-H or gardening
_____ Arts or crafts
_____ Chess or game clubs
_____ Music
_____ Other

What could we do at the school that could benefit the neighborhood?

_____

_____

When you think about your own skills, what are three things that you think you do best?

_____

_____

_____

What are three skills you would most like to learn?

_____

_____

Are there any skills you would like to teach or show others?

_____

_____

Are there some hobbies or special interests of yours that we have not covered?

_____

_____

How often do you go outside the neighborhood to have fun (in a week)?

Once a week or less _____ 2 to 4 times _____ Every day _____

Where do you go? _____

What kinds of new places or activities would you like to see in the neighborhood?

_____

_____

Are you part of any group that gets together on a regular basis? What are they?

_____

_____

Are you currently employed? _____

Which shift? _____

Is there any product or service related to your work that could be sold in the neighborhood?

_____

Should we let you know about our next meeting or activity? _____

Would you be interested in interviewing others? _____

Name: _____

Address: _____

Phone: _____

Interviewer's Name: _____

Date: _____

United Neighbors, Inc.
Paul Fessler
808 Harrison Street
Davenport, IA 52803
(536) 322-7363

Source: From Kretzmann, J., McKnight, J., and Sheehan, G. (1997). *A Guide to Capacity Inventories: Mobilizing the Community Skills of Local Residents.* Chicago: ACTA Publications; ABCD Institute. Davenport, IA: United Neighbors, Inc. Used with permission.

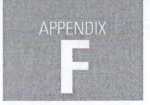

Early Detection Procedures

Early Detection Tips and Tools: Health Screening Guidelines and Resources

Put Your Plan in Motion

Daily, Monthly, and Yearly Checks

Learn what is normal for you, and to recognize important changes. There are many things you can do to detect problems early. These actions involve some "detective work" on your part—detective work called self-inspection. Self-inspection means that you monitor your own body and the way it's working. This helps you to learn what is normal for you, and to recognize important changes.

Your detective work involves three different types of self-inspection:

- **Every Day** Do quick checks of the way your body looks and feels, and the way it's functioning.
- **Monthly** Perform more thorough, overall self-exams. If you have a spouse or significant other, you can do some of these for each other.
- **Every 1–5 Years** Talk to your doctor about medical exams and screenings recommended every 1–5 years, based on your age and other risk factors.

You'll need to see the doctor for some of these tests. However, some may be available at low or no cost through early detection screenings at the worksite, community health fairs, or public health departments.

Do It for Life!

Remember, it's important that you play an active role in your early detection plan. Your doctor is very knowledgeable about diagnosing diseases and recommending treatments. But you will most likely be the first to recognize any changes. After all, only you know what's normal for your body.

Putting these three strategies into practice can ensure the earliest detection and fastest treatment of serious health problems. Doing them could save your life!

Use Reminders—Don't Forget!

Use this list to jog your memory. If you have a reminder card or copy of this list, hang it in the shower or on the bathroom door. Write reminders in your calendar. Seeing and acting on these reminders may save your life—or someone else's!

- Monitor yourself in the ways listed on these pages daily, monthly, and every 1–5 years.
- Use one or more self-care books to follow up on any symptoms.
- Consider your common sense or "gut" feelings when making medical decisions.
- Work with your doctor on early detection strategies and handling of problems.

Every Day

After you wake up, look in the mirror.

- Does your skin look healthy?
- Do your eyes look clear and alert?
- Look inside your mouth. Use your finger to feel around your gums and tongue for any sores. Note how your mouth and tongue look and feel.

Keep track of your bowel and bladder habits.

- Do you go more or less than normal?
- Any unusual color or appearance to your urine or stools?

Examine your feelings, energy level, and your body overall.

- If you don't feel your best, how long have you felt this way?
- Is there any pattern?

Examine your lifestyle choices.

- Are you eating foods high in nutrients and fiber, and low in fat and sodium most of the time?
- Are you getting 30 minutes of vigorous walking or some other aerobic activity at least 3 times each week?

- Are you getting 7–8 hours of sleep each night?
- Do you always wear your seat belt when traveling?
- Do you limit alcohol intake to fewer than 2 drinks per day?
- Are you safety conscious?
- Does your sexual conduct help you to avoid communicable diseases and unwanted pregnancy?
- Do you avoid the use of tobacco and other dangerous substances?
- Do you wash your hands regularly to avoid getting and spreading infections?

Every Month

Once per month, undress and observe your body in the mirror. Look at your skin color and texture from head to toe. Don't forget to check hidden areas (e.g., scalp, back, behind legs).

Look for areas of:

- Bruising or unusual colors
- Abnormal growths
- Changes in freckles or moles
- Unusual lumps

Reflect on how you've felt over the past month.

- Any unusual patterns in feelings, thoughts, relationships, and/or actions?

Weigh yourself and pinch your skin at the chest, waist, and thigh. Record and keep track of your results.

- Did you pinch more than 1 inch anywhere?
- Any unusual fluctuations in weight?

Women:

- Do a breast self-examination.
- Keep a record of the dates of your menstrual cycle and any associated problems.

Men:

- Do a testicular self-examination.

You can learn how to do self-exams of the breasts, testicles, and skin from self-care books, training programs, your doctor, and other health professionals.

Every 1–5 Years

Work with your doctor and use all available resources to create a schedule of recommended screenings and exams. Be sure to take into consideration your gender, age, current health status, and any existing risk factors (e.g., family history). These tests and exams should be performed every 1–5 years and may include:

- History and physical exam
- Health risk assessment
- Blood pressure
- Cholesterol, glucose, and other blood tests
- Urinalysis
- Vision and hearing

If you are over 50 you may be at increased risk for colorectal cancer and should consider digital rectal exam, fecal occult blood test (FOBT), and/or sigmoidoscopy.

For the early detection of prostate cancer, men over 50 should discuss PSA tests (prostate-specific antigen) with their doctor.

In addition, women should talk to their doctor about clinical breast exams, mammograms, and Pap tests.

Remember

You may be at increased risk for certain conditions if:

- You have a personal or family history of certain health problems
- Your lifestyle increases your risk (e.g., HIV/AIDS, hepatitis)

If you are considered high risk, you may need certain tests earlier and/or more often. Talk with your doctor about the tests you need and how often, based on your risks. Be sure to ask about immunizations you may need, too.

From: *Early Detection: Tips and Tools.* (2002). HPN Worldwide, Inc. Used with permission.

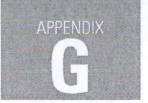

Community Risk Estimation

Harriet H. Imrey, Ph.D. *

Community risk estimation is a natural outgrowth of individual health appraisal. It depends upon the same basic sciences of public health—epidemiology and biostatistics—and can be done with more or less attention to the basic rules of evidence and statistical rigor. Barring serious biases in the selection of risk factors and relative risks for the model, a community risk appraisal is likely to be more accurate than an individual appraisal because one can use the law of large numbers as a security blanket.

We are hearing more about community risk estimation in public health circles than we used to. Risk reduction programs in the public sector must demonstrate an effect upon public health to justify public support. Community risk estimation is exactly what it says: an estimate. It is a way of projecting efficacy of risk reduction without waiting for years to demonstrate efficacy (or lack of it).

Appraising the health of a community can also be a source of civic pride if the appraisal is good, or a spur to action if it is not. It is easy to imagine: communities bidding for new industries on the grounds of a demonstrably healthy workforce. It is also easy to imagine the new industry listening to the argument, because we already know that a healthier workforce is a cheaper workforce.

Risk estimation can also be a useful means of needs assessment for program development, for public relations, or for policy decisions. It provides a tool

*Occupational Health Strategies, Inc., Charlottesville, VA, and Greenstone Healthcare Solutions, Kalamazoo, MI. Reprinted with the permission of Harriet H. Imrey, Ph.D., and the Society of Prospective Medicine. This paper appeared in the *Proceedings of the 21st Annual Meeting of the Society of Prospective Medicine,* 1986, pp. 8–11. Revised version, 1995.

for simulating the results of any number of health policy options in terms of deaths postponed or diseases prevented.

Community risk estimation can be used for business purposes. Private vendors of health risk appraisal instruments have already discovered the marketing potential for cost-effectiveness projections following worksite wellness programs—in this case, the individual company is the community of interest.

Before giving you a choice of several methods for estimating community risk, I would like to review some of the reasons for approaching this issue carefully. The bottom line for risk estimation in the community is calculating the population attributable risk proportion (PARP)—the percentage of deaths due to a particular risk factor—then multiplying this percentage by the number of deaths in the community. The only parameters you need to calculate this figure are the proportion of the population with the risk factor and the relative risk of death or disease for people who have the factor compared to those who do not:

$$PARP = \frac{p(RR - 1)}{1 + p(RR - 1)}$$

This is very straightforward when you are working with one binary risk factor (people have it or they don't). The only complications arise when you want to use more than one risk factor or a risk factor with several gradients of risk, such as heavy smoking, light smoking, and nonsmoking. Unfortunately, we almost always want to do it thus way, and have to cope with the complexities.

The simplest example is a data set based on two risk factors, where the data show no confounding and no interaction. For our purposes, "no confounding" means that people who have or do not have risk factor A have equal probabilities of having risk factor B; A and B are not associated. "No interaction" means that the relative risk of B is the same whether or not the person has risk factor A (see **Table 1**).

TABLE 1
PARP Example of *Two* Risk Factors with No Confounding and No Interaction

	N	p	r	d	RR
AB	1,000	0.10	0.04	40	4.0
A$\bar{\text{B}}$	3,000	0.30	0.02	60	2.0
$\bar{\text{A}}$B	1,500	0.15	0.02	30	2.0
$\bar{\text{A}}\bar{\text{B}}$	4,500	0.45	0.01	45	1.0
Total	10,000		0.0175	175	

(Continued)

TABLE 1
(*Continued*)

Population Attributable Risk Proportion (PARP)

$$= r \frac{(\text{Total}) - r(\overline{A}\,\overline{B})}{r(\text{Total})} = \frac{0.0175 - 0.01}{0.0175} = 42.86\%$$

or

$$1 - \frac{1}{\sum pRR} = 1 - \frac{1}{0.10(4) + 0.30(2) = 0.15(2) = 0.45(1)}$$

$$= 1 - \frac{1}{1.75} = 42.86\%$$

One variable at a time:

	N	p	r	d	RR
A	4,000	0.40	0.025	100	2.0
$\overline{A}$	6,000	0.60	0.0125	75	1.0
	10,000 I		0.0175	175	

$$PARP(A) = 28.57\%$$

	N	p	r	d	RR
B	2,500	0.25	0.028	70	2.0
$\overline{B}$	7,500	0.75	0.014	105	1.0
	10,000		0.0175	175	

$$PARP(B) = 20.0\%$$

Total Population Attributable Risk Proportion

$$= 1 - \pi[1 - PARP(X)] = 1 - (1 - 28.57\%)(1 - 20.0\%) = 42.86\%$$

The easiest way to look at population attributable risk, when you have a complete set of data such as this, is to look at the death rate among the group that has neither risk factor, and see by what proportion the total death rate would go down if everyone were at that low risk level. In this case, it would be 42.86%. In the real world, we don't have this information for the community we are working with, so we have to make the first great leap of faith: We assume that a relative risk represents some sort of biological truth that applies to the world at large, and that unknown risk factors are not busily confounding our data source. Then we can go ahead and use these relative risk figures with prevalence data from our own community.

Again, back in the real world, we might not know anything about the joint distribution of the risk factors and know only what proportion of people have factor A and what proportion have factor B. In this case only, we have the option of working with one variable at a time. The total PARP, calculated by combining the PARP figures for the two variables and using the last formula for Table 1, is the same as that calculated with the first formula. One important thing to notice here is that the PARP figures cannot be added together, because the same death would be accounted for more than once: Your community risk estimate would look odd, if you promised to reduce the death rate by 150%.

The next example shows the effects of confounding: What happens when your risk factors are not distributed independently in the original data sources (Table 2). The important thing here is that the relative risks you would be using are not the true (un-confounded) relative risks: part of the effect measured for factor A is due to the larger proportion of B people in the A category, and vice versa. Both relative risks are overestimates of the true relative risk—that is, the risk after adjustment for confounding. The result in this case is an overestimate of the community attributable risk by 18%.

TABLE 2
PARP Example of Two Risk Factors with Confounding and No Interaction [$P(B|A) = 0.15$, not 0.10]

Confounding: The likelihood of possessing risk factor B is different depending on whether or not the person possesses factor A (e.g., a sedentary person may be somewhat more likely to smoke than a jogger).

	N	p	r	d	RR
AB	1,500	0.15	0.04	60	4.0
A$\bar{\text{B}}$	2,500	0.25	0.02	50	2.0
$\bar{\text{A}}$B	1,000	0.10	0.02	20	2.0
$\bar{\text{A}}\bar{\text{B}}$	5,000	0.50	0.01	50	1.0
Total	10,000		0.018	180	

$$PARP = \frac{0.018 - 0.01}{0.018} = 44.44\%$$

One variable at a time:

	N	p	r	d	RR
A	4,000	0.40	0.0275	110	2.36
$\bar{\text{A}}$	6,000	0.60	0.0117	70	1.0
	10,000		0.018	180	

(Continued)

TABLE 2
(*Continued*)

$$PARP(A) = 35.0\%$$

	N	p	r	d	RR
B	2,500	0.25	0.320	80	2.41
$\overline{B}$	7,500	0.75	0.0133	100	1.0
	10,000		0.0180	180	

$$PARP(B) = 26.06\%$$

$$1 - (1 - 0.35)(1 - 0.2606) = 51.94\% \text{ (not right)}$$

Table 3 shows confounding and interaction at the same time. If the only information you have is two separate relative risks and the population prevalence for each, your community attributable risk estimate will be inaccurate.

The point of this somewhat tedious review is to demonstrate that you will almost never have enough information to estimate community risk correctly for more than a very few variables at a time, because you need to be sure that the relative risks have been adjusted for confounding, that interactions have been accounted for, and that you know the joint distribution of all risk factors in your population. The latter procedure becomes especially tedious when more than very few risk factors are involved.

The catch to this methodological warning is that these conditions cannot be met with relative risk data available at this point in time. The choices are to do nothing—even though many of us have a real need for estimates of community risk—or to proceed very carefully with the best data we can get, but make no unwarranted claims about the precision of the estimates. By supporting the use of individual health risk appraisals, we have already decided to take the latter course. All of us are barefoot empiricists who jump into applications based on epidemiologic evidence that usually falls far short of proof. What we do is make decisions on the weight of the evidence, as a jury in a civil court must do. If we waited for "beyond a reasonable doubt," we would still hesitate about advocating any form of health education or health promotion activities.

We have just reviewed the methodological reasons why community risk estimation should not be attempted. However, here are some directions to accomplish such an estimation. Table 4 shows what to do if the only facts you know are the proportion of the population with each of several risk factors, and the relative risks that apply to that factor. You have to have faith that the risk factors are distributed independently in the study population that the relative risks came from and in your own community, and faith will

TABLE 3
PARP Example of Two Risk Factors with Confounding and Interaction [*RR*(AB) = 5, not 4]

Interaction: The effect on mortality of risk factor B is greater if the person also possesses risk factor A (e.g., a sedentary lifestyle may be more hazardous among smokers than among nonsmokers).

	N	p	r	d	RR
AB	1,500	0.15	0.05	75	5.0
A$\bar{\text{B}}$	2,500	0.25	0.02	50	2.0
$\bar{\text{A}}$B	1,000	0.10	0.02	20	2.0
$\bar{\text{A}}\bar{\text{B}}$	5,000	0.50	0.01	50	1.0
Total	10,000		0.0195	195	

$$PARP = \frac{0.0195 - 0.01}{0.0195} = 48.72\%$$

One variable at a time:

	N	p	r	d	RR
A	4,000	0.40	0.03125	125	2.68
$\bar{\text{A}}$	6,000	0.60	0.0117	70	1.0
	10,000		0.0195	195	

$$PARP(A) = 40.2\%$$

	N	p	r	d	RR
B	2,500	0.25	0.038	95	2.85
$\bar{\text{B}}$	7,500	0.75	0.0133	100	1.0
	10,000		0.0195	195	

$$PARP(B) = 31.62\%$$

$$1 - (1 - 0.402)(1 - 0.3162) = 59.11\% \textbf{ (not right)}$$

TABLE 4
Risk Estimation Process with Community Prevalence Rates for Individual Risk Factors

---

What You Know:

1. Number (or rate) of deaths

2. Relative risks (RR) for one or more risk factors

3. Community prevalence rates (p) for one or more risk factors

What You Believe:

Risk factors are distributed independently in the population and there are no interactions among the relative risks.

What You Do:

1. For *one* risk factor:

$$PARP = \frac{p(RR - 1)}{1 + p(RR - 1)}$$

Deaths that may be postponable = number of deaths $\times$ *PARP*

2. For *one or more* risk factors:

$$PARP = 1 - \pi[1 - PARP(X)]$$

For example, if the *PARP* for smoking is 30% and the *PARP* for inactivity is 20%, the total attributable risk proportion is $1 - (1 - 0.30)(1 - 0.20) = 44\%$.

---

be less strenuous if you don't try to account for factors you know to be related—such as relative weight, blood pressure, and exercise—in the same model. No one can force you to be sensible about it, because the equations don't care one way or the other.

You can do a much better job of community risk estimation if you know the joint prevalence distribution of all the risk factors in your model, and if you have faith that the relative risks you use are "pure" ones—that is, relative risks adjusted for confounding or derived from a multivariate model. You might even have relative risks for interactions. In practice, if you know the joint prevalence of risk factors, you probably know the composite relative risk of each member of your community sample. You have a choice of equations. Table 5 shows the computation of the population attributable risk proportion for grouped data. If you have a computerized data set with risk factor prevalence survey data, it is more efficient to use this formula.

$$PARP = 1 - \frac{N}{\sum CCR}$$

TABLE 5
Risk Estimation Process with Community Prevalence Rates for Combinations of Risk Factors

What You Know:
1. Number (or rate) of deaths
2. Relative risks (RR) for one or more risk factors
3. Community prevalence rate (p) for each combination of risk factors, from a population survey or from risk appraisals
What You Believe:
The risk factors are not distributed independently, but you believe that the relative risks in your model do not interact with one another except in those cases where you have identified a separate relative risk for the categories where interactions take place.
What You Do:
$$PARP = 1 - \frac{1}{\sum pCRR}$$ where p is the proportion of the population with a particular combination of risk factors, and CRR is the composite relative risk for that particular combination (i.e., the product of all relative risks for each separate risk factor).

The composite relative risk for a community (relative to what the community would be like if every resident reduced all reducible risk factors) is always the inverse of the population unattributable risk proportion, just as the composite relative risk for an individual is the inverse of his or her own unattributable risk proportion. Given this fact, it is easy to compare two states or communities directly, and make inappropriate comparisons. One can imagine health educators arguing indefinitely over a model that asserted that Montana is exactly 37.5% healthier than Arkansas. A large lawsuit over a suspected environmental contaminant centered on the argument, based on this methodology, that the cancer rate in the affected community, after accounting for other *known* risk factors, was even lower than the cancer rate in the control community, proving that no excess cases could be blamed on a carcinogen in the water supply.

In the future, we will see a growing number of examples of this sort, and we can expect to see more people estimating community risk based on more accurate models. In the meantime, it is necessary to be very cautious about creating synthetic models from very crude data, but that doesn't mean it can't be done. We haven't even touched on questions of selecting all-cause mortality models versus summing over individual causes of death, although the former

TABLE 6
Risk Estimation Process with Risk Factor Prevalence Data for Each Subject

> **What You Know:**
>
> 1. Number (or rate) of deaths
>
> 2. Relative risks (*RR*) for one or more risk factors
>
> 3. Risk factor prevalence data for each individual in your population sample
>
> **What You Believe:**
>
> The relative risks in your model do not interact with one another except in those cases where you have a separate relative risk for the categories where interactions take place.
>
> **What You Do:**
>
> $$PARP = 1 - \frac{N}{\sum CRR}$$
>
> where *CRR* is the composite relative risk (product of individual relative risks) for each individual in your sample of *N* people.

is generally more conservative. We also haven't considered inaccuracies based upon different risk factor prevalence distributions in different age groups: The safest procedure is to use proportions and relative risks for the narrowest age groups for which data are available. We haven't talked about additive versus multiplicative models, although similar techniques have been derived for additive models. Failing to consider any one of these issues can make your community risk estimates less accurate. However, if you back off because the procedure is complicated, you will miss the opportunity to get some very interesting and useful information that may be only a little bit in error.

In summary, take whatever information you have, add any information you can reasonably get, and take full advantage of every single piece of it. If you have access to your state's Risk Factor Prevalence Survey database, or to a file of computerized health risk appraisals, you are ready to do community risk appraisal with a fair degree of accuracy for a very small investment.

Technical Notation: How to Read the Tables

The probability notation used in the examples may be unfamiliar to many readers, but is not nearly so complicated as it looks. The A and B stand for two different risk factors, such as smoking and obesity. A bar over the top is a negative symbol: It means that the risk factor is not present. In Table 1, the second row that starts out with $A\bar{B}$ stands for that part of the population of

10,000 people who have risk factor A (they smoke), but do not have risk factor B (they are not overweight). The number (N) of people in that category is 3,000; the category's proportion (p) of the total is 0.30.

The rate (r) of death is 0.02, meaning that $3000 \times 0.02 = 60$ people in the category will die (d). The relative risk (RR) is the death rate in that category compared to the death rate among people who do not have either of the risk factors (the row that starts with $\overline{A}\overline{B}$), so the relative risk for category $A\overline{B}$ is $0.02/0.01 = 2$. It takes a little bit of time to figure out any new notation, but using this one can be very time-saving when communicating complex numerical examples.

Index